...ED ULTIMATE
NUTRITION

The Ultimate Nutrition Guide for Joint and Arthritic Conditions

Zoe Hellman Bsc SRD

Emerald Guides
www.emeraldpublishing.co.uk

Emerald Guides
Brighton BN2 4EG

ISBN 9781847161253

Printed by GN Press, Essex

Cover design by Donna McCann

Whilst every effort has been made to ensure that the information
contained within this book is correct at the time of going to press, the
author and publisher can take no responsibility for the errors or
omissions contained within.

Contents

Introduction

This book offers a comprehensive guide to equip those affected by joint and arthritic conditions with a sound and trusted foundation of nutritional advice and support. It aims to empower readers with the understanding and practical knowledge to optimise health and well being through evidence based nutritional therapy.

Based on the latest research and practice, this book covers the importance of nutrition and how to apply key principles to the diet. Part 1 offers targeted advice for those suffering from; rheumatoid arthritis, osteoarthritis and gout. Part 2 offers useful chapters to pick and choose from – simply read those most useful.

In some chapters, sample day's intakes are given to help illustrate suggested dietary techniques. They are not nutritionally balanced menus. Anyone wishing to implement any dietary techniques should consult with a registered dietitian to ensure that their diet is nutritionally balanced whilst meeting their individual needs.

Always consult a registered dietitian or health professional before engaging with any kind nutritional therapy and again if problems persist.

Part One
Joint and Arthritic Conditions

Chapter One

Rheumatoid Arthritis

Rheumatoid arthritis (RA)

RA is an autoimmune, progressive disease. The disease itself is characterized by 'flare-ups' and periods of remission, the length of which can be varying. It has both localised and systemic effects, which means that the disease's inflammatory nature impacts on both musculoskeletal areas that are directly affected, commonly the peripheral joints i.e. those at the extremities for example the ankles or wrists, and the body as a whole, with many other organs and hence body functions affected.

When someone is suffering a 'flare-up' the body produces lots of internal signals to increase inflammation, which is why the whole body is affected in RA and not just the area affected.

Common symptoms include; joint pain in the feet, wrists and hands, which may be accompanied by swelling and morning stiffness. It is also very common to experience fever, daily tiredness and low mood with periods of extreme fatigue. As the disease progresses, joint damage can occur due to the periodical cycle of; inflammation, damage and repair, which may impact on physical mobility and strength.

Although the triggers for the development of the disease are largely unknown and much more research is needed to understand it better, it is thought that a genetic susceptibility plays a role.

At the moment, there is no cure for RA. Treatment aims to suppress the progress, minimise frequency of flare-ups and negative health impacts of the disease and its treatment.

Common conditions associated with the systemic impact that RA has include; fever, loss of appetite, tiredness, weakness, swollen lymph nodes, anaemia, dry eyes, fibrosis of the lungs, fluid in the chest cavity, vasculitis and GI and kidney problems.

Some RA sufferers may also experience 'rheumatoid cachexia'. The term cachexia (kak ex ee a) describes a complex state of weight loss and under-nutrition. Cachexia comes from the Greek words Kakos, meaning 'bad' and Hexis, meaning 'condition'.

The weight loss associated with cachexia tends to see losses of both muscle and fat. The weight loss driven by rheumatoid cachexia is very different to weight loss through diet or exercise where the majority of weight loss is fat. It is caused primarily by changes in metabolism associated with the inflammatory process of RA, sometimes in combination with a reduction in dietary intake due to the side effects of the disease.

Changes in metabolism in rheumatoid cachexia

The bodies' normal process of metabolism (the breakdown and usage of the different nutrients) can be affected by RA causing the body to become 'hypermetabolic'. When the body is hypermetabolic there are some key changes in the breakdown and usage of nutrients:

- Changes in fat metabolism – The stores of fat in the body are broken down much more quickly and the rate that the body stores fat is reduced. This means that overall stores of body fat are decreased.

- Changes in protein metabolism – The human body does not have any stores or reserves of protein. This is because all the protein within the body has important functions to fulfil. Most of the protein within the body is used to make up muscle, but protein also plays a major role in the immune system. Cachexia causes the breakdown of these vital body proteins and reduces the generation of new proteins. When the body breaks down its own proteins, a process known as catabolism, this can have effects on body weight, muscle strength, organ function and the immune system.
- Changes in carbohydrate metabolism – The body is not able to use carbohydrate as efficiently as should. This inefficiency could account for around 300kcals a day of lost energy.

In addition to these changes in metabolism, hypermetabolism also increases Basic Metabolic Rate (BMR). BMR is the rate at which food (calories) are used up. This means that the body's overall nutritional requirements are increased. So, despite eating a seemingly sufficient diet, weight may be lost because the body is burning calories much faster than normal.

Figure 1.1 illustrates the hierarchy of metabolism – the way that different food groups are used as energy in the body. Figure 1.1 shows that the first source of energy the body will naturally use is carbohydrates. During periods of reduced dietary intake or more specifically reduced carbohydrate intake, body proteins and then fat stores are called upon for energy to fuel the body. In a state of hypermetabolism, these energy sources are called upon more quickly to ensure there is sufficient fuel for the body.

Figure 1.1 Hierarchy of metabolism

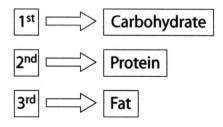

If the way different food groups are used for energy is considered, it is clear that in the first instance, having sufficient carbohydrates is crucial to help protect against the breakdown of body proteins and fat stores.

Due to these changes in metabolism, is can be very difficult to reverse weight loss associated with RA. Trying to *minimise* the loss of weight and *protect* body proteins and fat stores should be a major goal.

The effect of losses of body proteins

The disease process in RA can cause the loss of fat stores and body proteins. The majority of body proteins are muscles. It is commonly believed that when muscle is lost it is from the muscles used for mobility and strength such the arms and legs. However, when muscle is lost, it can be lost from any muscle within the body, including those in the heart and lungs.

The main role of the lungs is to inhale air to gather oxygen for the blood. The main role of the heart is to pump blood around every part of the body. When muscle from the heart and lungs is lost these essential processes can be affected.

An under-nourished heart;

- Has reduced strength to pump blood around the body
- Pumps smaller amounts of blood at one time

Under-nourished lungs;
- Have a reduced ability to inhale air
- Have a reduced amount of air that can be inhaled
- Have a reduced overall ability to get oxygen into the blood

RA and it's treatment increases:	Possible reasons why:	Useful information can be found in these chapters:
The risk of being under-nourished	Due to hypermetabolism, small appetite, under-nourished tiredness, low mood and mobility problems impacting on food intake Due to adopting a 'self-help' diet	Joint and arthritic conditions and being Fact vs Fiction section in this chapter

Continued

The risk of being overweight	Due to reduced ability to get active and side-effects of some RA common treatments	Joint and arthritic conditions and being overweight Medications
Long term health risk of developing cardiovascular disease	Due to the inflammatory nature of RA	Cardiovascular health
Long term health risk of developing osteoporosis	Due to common treatments for RA	Medications

Key dietary manipulations important for those suffering from RA

Nutritional therapy can help to minimise the effects of the disease, its treatment and long term health risks. The key dietary manipulations that can help RA sufferers are:

- Being a healthy weight and well nourished. Please refer to the chapters; 'how to assess nutritional status,' relevant chapters on being overweight or under-nourished and 'a well balanced healthy diet'.
- Correct nutritional deficiencies caused by the disease process or treatment. Please see relevant information in this chapter and refer to chapter 'medications'.
- Ensure a cardiovascular and bone healthy diet, Please refer to chapters; 'cardiovascular health' and 'medications'
- Promote anti-inflammation
- Decrease joint damage

The inflammatory process and antioxidants

The reactions involved in natural life, such as breathing and metabolism create, amongst many others, waste products called free radicals.

Free radicals are highly reactive molecules that can damage sensitive tissues within the human body, such as DNA or cell walls. Free radicals also increase the risk of developing cardiovascular disease and can exacerbate joint damage, particularly if inflammation is present.

Antioxidants, which are certain vitamin and minerals in the diet, help to protect the body against damage from free radicals. Normally, the body can handle free radicals, but if antioxidants are low or unavailable, or if the production of free radicals becomes excessive, damage to the body can occur.

Environmental factors such as pollution, radiation and cigarette smoke can create free radicals. Free radical damage is known to accumulate with age, so the older we get – the more important it is to have sufficient antioxidant protection. Inflammation increases the generation of free radicals, so for those with inflammatory diseases, antioxidant protection is even more vital.

The constancy and unavoidability of free radical production imposes a great importance on a diet rich in antioxidants. The human body has a fundamental daily need for antioxidants. Antioxidants:

- Form a physical barrier against free radicals, preventing access to delicate body cells

- Absorb free radicals by acting as 'scavengers'
- Neutralise free radicals making them unable to cause any damage
- Help decrease the initial production of free radicals

The threat within the body between an imbalance of free radicals and antioxidants is a constant one. A constant and sufficient intake of antioxidants is therefore needed to help prevent free radical damage.

Antioxidants come in a variety of forms and include; vitamin C, vitamin E, vitamin A and selenium. The best way to consume sufficient antioxidants is to eat a wide range of fruit and vegetables daily (please refer to the chapter 'a healthy well balanced diet' for more information). Antioxidants are particularly abundant in deep coloured fruit and vegetables, such as spinach, carrots, broccoli, sweet potatoes, peppers, tomatoes, mangos, apricots and oranges.

A historical approach

The human body's nutritional needs, rooted in our ancient nutritional programming, are thought to be outmatched by contemporary living and dietary habits. Humans have been evolving for more than 2 million years developing partly though the transition from fibreous roughage to intakes of higher quality foods. Intakes of plant derived antioxidants of Palaeolithic humans (Iron Age) is thought to be many times greater than currently population intakes.

Vitamin C
Palaeolithic Diets: 604mg
Modern Diets: 59–115mg

Vitamin E
Palaeolithic Diets: 33mg
Modern Diets: 5.2–5.5 mg

The adaptation of the human body has been impossible to match the rapid advancement of agriculture. Some say that there is a key dispute between physiological need for antioxidants and the content in traditional Western diets.

Routine supplementation of antioxidants has not proven to be beneficial for sufferers of RA in terms of symptom relief. However, sufficient intakes of antioxidants is certainly needed for long term health, so a varied and abundant intake of fruit and vegetables and wholegrain foods is advisable.

The inflammatory process and iron

People with RA are at an increased risk of developing iron-deficiency anaemia. Iron-deficiency anaemia is caused by a lack of iron. It is a condition where there are too few red blood cells, or insufficient haemoglobin (the element that carries oxygen within the red blood cell). This can cause feelings of tiredness and breathlessness.

People with RA are at risk of this condition, as its inflammatory nature suppresses the production of haemoglobin. It is thought that iron is needed elsewhere by inflamed tissues, so the body prioritises iron for this function as opposed to haemoglobin production. Research has found that people with RA tend to consume low levels of iron in their diets, further compounding this situation. In addition, some medications used to treat RA also increase the risk of iron-deficiency anaemia.

There is no evidence to show that routine iron supplementation is needed, but some people may require supplementation if they are known to be depleted. Ensuring a regular and sufficient intake of iron in the diet is important for RA sufferers. Discussing supplementation needs with a qualified health care professional is advisable.

What is iron?

Iron is a mineral and is an important part of a healthy diet because it helps red blood cells transport oxygen around the body.

Whilst most men eat enough iron, many women are not eating enough. Recent surveys suggest that 25% of women in the UK eat much less iron than their daily requirements and that women are consuming significantly less iron than men, which is rather worrying as a women's daily requirements are actually higher than a man's, primarily due to losses associated with the menstrual cycle.

Iron in the diet can come from both meat and non-meat sources. The iron from meat (called heam-iron) is quite easily absorbed by the body, but the iron from non-meat sources (called non-heam iron) is not. The recommended daily amount for an adult is 8.7mg a day for men and 14.8mg a day for women. Meat is the best source of iron, because it tends to contain a lot of it and in a form that is easily absorbed by the body. Non- meat sources of iron include:

- Beans and pulses
- Dark green leafy vegetables such as watercress, broccoli, curly kale, spring greens and okra
- Bread
- Wholegrains (like brown rice)
- Fortified breakfast cereals

To help the body absorb iron from food, getting enough vitamin C in the diet is important. This is because vitamin C aids the absorption of iron from food. Aiming to have some fruit or vegetables or a glass of fruit juice at mealtimes can help aid iron absorption. Good sources of vitamin C include peppers, oranges, fruit juices, sweet potatoes and kiwi fruit.

Also, cutting down on tea and coffee could help to improve iron levels in the body too. This is because components found in tea and coffee, called polyphenols, can inhibit the absorption of iron from food, so avoid drinking these an hour before and an hour after a meal.

A word of caution

Red meat:

Red meat is a great source of protein and other essential nutrients like zinc, selenium and B vitamins. It is also one of the best sources of easily absorbed iron.

However, red meat needs to be limited (such as beef, pork and lamb) and processed meats (bacon, salami, corned beef and some sausages) avoided if possible. This is because there is strong scientific evidence that red and processed meats increases risk of developing bowel cancer. In fact, there is no amount of processed meat that can be confidently shown *not* to increase the risk.

Try to limit red meat to less than 500g cooked weight (about 700–750g raw weight) a week. For example having; one 8oz rump steak, a portion of Bolognese and 2 slices of ham – would take someone to their maximum weekly intake of red meat. Check the weight of red meat intake by looking at food labels.

Inflammation and omega-3 fatty acids

People with chronic inflammatory processes, as seen in those with RA, may benefit from supplementation of omega-3 fatty acids. For more information on omega-3 fatty acids, what they are and where to find them please refer to this chapter.

It is possible that omega-3 fatty acids help to reduce inflammatory processes by decreasing the production of inflammatory messages and signals within the body. Specifically for those with RA, there has been much research into the possible effect of supplementation.

Although many studies have not seen an improvement in disease progression with omega-3 supplementation, some have seen improvements in pain and tenderness of joints and duration of morning stiffness. However, the debate about *how much* is needed to bring these positive benefits continues. It is thought that there is a threshold below which would not bring any benefit and above which would start to see benefit. Supplementation has been proven to be needed to be over an extended period of time. Some studies have found modest benefits after supplementation of an average of 3–6g EPA+DHA daily over a continuous period of at least 12 weeks. This level of intake would be very difficult to achieve via the diet alone.

Although this may seem like a piece of advice that can be easily followed to improve joint tenderness and morning stiffness, the safety of this level of high dose supplementation long term is not yet know. It is therefore recommended that people suffering from RA aim for a healthy level of oily fish intake and do not take high dose supplements until there is more evidence that it is safe to do so. Discussing supplementation with a qualified health professional may be beneficial.

Other oils that may offer benefits in RA

It is thought that other oils, such as evening primrose, hemp, blackcurrant seed and borage seed (rich in a type of fatty acid called GLA) may benefit people with OA and RA, as GLA is said to have anti-inflammatory properties. GLA is an essential fatty acid (EFA) in the omega-6 family, found primarily in plant-based oils. For more information on omega-6 and omega-3 oils please refer to the chapter 'omega-3 fatty acids'.

Initial studies have looked at supplementing high dose GLA (at around 1.4g a day) for at least 6 months and found it may help to reduce pain and joint swelling in RA sufferers. However, it is still early days and more research is needed to understand the ideal dose of GLA and whether there is any safety issues supplementing at these high doses. For example it is known that GLA may increase the possibility of miscarriage.

Studies that have looked specifically at Evening Primrose Oil (EPO) have shown that they may help to relieve inflammation. EPO needs to be taken for a minimum of 3–6 months before positive effects can be seen. And, EPO needs to be taken continuously in order for any benefits to continue.

Spirulina, otherwise known as Blue-Green algae is rich in proteins, vitamins, minerals and GLA. It is thought that spirulina may help to reduce inflammation. Supplements like this one derived from seaweed, have been claimed to help improve pain and stiffness. However, because of the potential for side effects and interactions with medications, supplements should be taken only under the supervision of a qualified health professional and should not be taken during pregnancy because they may be harmful. At the moment the research is still too sparse and insufficient to be able to provide advice on the safety or effectiveness of algae derived supplements.

Olive oil is also known to possess anti-inflammatory properties, but again more research is needed to understand its potential impact on OA and RA. It would seem prudent to switch from using spreads that are made from vegetable oils or using vegetable oils in cooking, to using olive oil and olive oil based spreads.

Fact or fiction – nutrition and RA

I have met many people who have adopted 'alternative' nutritional advice from various unreliable sources. The advice from these sources was trusted, as it was presented in such a way that suggested the principles were safe and well researched. However, these 'alternative' diets are often strict, eliminating essential food groups, and hence nutrients from the diet, or add in expensive supplements that are simply of no benefit. In addition advice from these sources can be expensive. The majority of alternative diets at best do not promote health and wellbeing and at worst compromise health and wellbeing.

It is well known that nutrition has a direct impact on health. There are many different 'alternative' diets that are promoted for people suffering from RA the claims of which can sometimes be confusing.

The episodic flare-ups seen in RA are easily attributed to external factors such as diet or lifestyle. This lends weight to many claims of certain faddy approaches. However, at the moment the triggers or episodic nature of RA is poorly understood.

It is absolutely understandable why ideas that simple dietary answers can help fight this complicated autoimmune disease, are very appealing. Claims are made that special diets, certain foods and supplements may help to cure or alleviate symptoms of RA, but most claims are unproven and could be harmful rather than helpful. There is however, a wealth of reliable scientific evidence which shows that a healthy, well balanced diet supports the human body for good health and wellbeing. For more information on a healthy well balanced diet please refer to this chapter.

Before starting any special diet or taking any RA remedy, it is important to discuss with a qualified health professional any evidence for effectiveness, any side-effects or possibly harmful interaction with prescription medicine.

How to spot a faddy, unproven dietary claim

- Does the diet ask for the elimination of a complete food group, such as dairy?
- Does the diet ask for the elimination of a list of certain foods?
- Does the diet have any potentially harmful effects?
- Does the diet use personal testimonies, instead of scientific evidence, to support it?
- Does the diet ask for expensive supplementations?

Vitamin and mineral supplementation

Vitamin and mineral supplementation is commonly advocated to those suffering from RA and it may be required in some people who suffer from proven deficiencies or are undergoing certain treatments guided by a health professional. However, there is no evidence that supplementing vitamins and minerals as a routine habit is needed or indeed has any positive effects for people with RA.

In fact, simply supplementing the diet with different vitamins and minerals without the guidance of a health professional could put health at risk. This is because the different vitamins and minerals work in synergy with each other. If there is an 'overdose' of one and a lack of the other, their functions are likely to be disrupted. And, taking too much of certain vitamins or minerals (particularly the fat soluble ones) can be unhealthy, as levels could build up in the body to 'toxic' levels.

Despite some media reports or sales pitches, research into supplementation with copper, zinc or selenium have found no proven significant benefits for those suffering from RA.

Vitamins and minerals

These are chemicals needed by the body, often in small quantities, to perform essential functions. Most can not be made by the body itself so are an essential part of a healthy well balanced diet.

Fat soluble vitamins – Vitamin A, D, K and E

This means they are found and stored in fats within the diet and the body. It is therefore possible that stores can be built up over a lifetime, meaning that there can be large stores within the body which could potentially become excessive if consumption exceeds need.

Water soluble vitamins – Vitamins B and C

This means they are found within foods containing water and that they are needed in frequent regular intakes, as any excess intakes are excreted in the urine. Therefore risk of deficiency is high for those with a lack of variety in the diet.

Fasting

Only very few studies have shown that fasting mildly reduces joint pain and swelling in RA, but these effects are only transient. As soon as normal diet is resumed, any minor benefits return very quickly. Fasting is a very high-risk approach to trying to alleviate RA symptoms.

Fasting is likely to have significant impacts on overall nutritional status and is not recommended as healthy or beneficial in any way.

Food intolerances and allergy

There is no evidence that people with RA have any higher rates of food allergy or intolerances compared with the general population.

A food intolerance is one which tends to have a mild reaction, indicating that the body has 'difficulty dealing with a particular food'. Symptoms commonly include; nausea, vomiting, diarrhoea, bloating and abdominal discomfort.

The human gut absorbs and deals with food antigens on a daily basis. An antigen is a substance that prompts the generation an immune response within the body, so a food antigen is a substance originating from food that triggers an immune response by the body. A food allergy is one which triggers an immune response, such as swelling of the tongue, lips and mouth, a rash and exacerbating inflammation in general.

For those suffering from chronic inflammatory conditions, including RA, avoiding exacerbation of the immune system is sensible.

It is thought that the gut (the part of the digestive system that absorbs food) may be affected by common medications used to treat RA, making it weaker and more likely to allow certain substances through its protection system (see page 67). Given that RA sufferers have changes in the regulation of inflammation and possible reduced immunity in the gut, there *may* be a greater risk of developing an allergy to certain foods. In very few, exceptional cases; exclusion diets have identified individuals in whom a specific food exacerbates RA symptoms.

Alcohol, pickles, citrus fruits, tomatoes, vinegars, bananas, chocolate, malt, onions, soy products, cane sugar, spices (cardamom, coriander, and mint), caffeine, certain vegetables, fizzy drinks, sugar, additives, preservatives and salt are claimed by personal accounts, to have an effect on RA symptoms. There has been some research into the effect of excluding these foods and in addition; dairy products, gluten-containing products, red meat and cereals – however none have shown any benefits generally for those with RA.

Some people may claim symptomatic benefit of excluding certain food groups or foods from their diet, however this benefit is likely to be subjective and not backed up by reliable, clinical results. It is believed that the placebo effect plays an extremely strong role in this area. In addition, RA sufferers could indeed feel benefits from changing their diet associated with weight loss or because their RA had gone into a remission phase at the same time.

> **There is no evidence that excluding food groups or certain food from the diet will bring significant symptomatic or health benefits to the general population suffering from RA**

Imposing unnecessary food restrictions may in fact be risky for people with RA. As it will have an impact on vitamin and mineral intake and antioxidant levels, which we know are so important to maintain health. Optimum advice is to avoid food restrictions and instead aim for a varied and well-balanced diet.

In order to identify a food allergy or intolerance, a similar process needs to occur: an elimination diet. An elimination diet is time consuming, often taking months to effectively complete and requires the careful guidance of a qualified health professional to ensure safety and accuracy. If it is thought that a certain food is exacerbating symptoms, full assessment and a food exclusion process needs to be undertaken together with a registered dietitian.

A word of warning

There are many 'food allergy' tests out there that claim to be able to diagnose from; a few drops of blood, strands of hair or a skin prick test of a range of foods for example. Being able to identify a true food allergy (and hence the only way to be able to find out what is going on, to be able to make the most effective changes to the diet) takes close and careful monitoring. Don't get fooled. The process of identifying a true food allergy is an extensive process that needs to be undertaken with a qualified health professional. If anybody claims otherwise, it's likely that they are trying to con people out of money. The consequences of listening to these 'experts in food allergy' may actually negatively affect health.

Herbal remedies

Despite sales claims there is very little scientific evidence that herbal remedies help alleviate symptoms of RA. In fact, there is very little scientific evidence to support the safety of taking herbal remedies. More research is needed to understand how these herbal remedies react with common RA medications (as they could affect efficacy and may have toxic effects) and whether these herbal remedies are safe to take at all.

Spices

Some spices including ginger, clove oil, garlic, turmeric and cumin have been claimed to help reduce inflammation in laboratory tests (in other words not tested on humans). However, there is no good quality scientific research that has tested the effects of spices on inflammation in humans let alone any potential effects on RA, so it should not be believed that they offer an effective treatment.

Aloe vera

Aloe is commonly used in external gels and creams to soothe and reduce inflammation. It is also available as a drink and some claim that it can have a positive effect on RA. However, the evidence does not show any promising benefits for taking aloe internally to treat or improve symptoms of RA.

Bromelain

Bromelain is also known as Ananas Comosus, and is a mixture of enzymes that help to digest protein, and is claimed to be able to reduce inflammation, swelling and pain. However, there is no good quality scientific evidence to support this theory.

CMO

CMO (otherwise known as cetyl myristoleate) is derived from beef tallow and is often promoted as a cure for OA and RA. However, there is no good quality scientific evidence to support its use, in fact it is potentially very dangerous as people are advised to stop taking their regular arthritis medications when on CMO.

MSM

MSM (otherwise known as methyl sulfonyl methane) is also claimed to be a 'cure' all for OA and RA. However, there is no good quality scientific evidence to support its use.

Devil's Claw

Devil's Claw is a supplement derived from an African desert plant called Devil's Claw. It is claimed to poses anti-inflammatory properties. However little research has been carried out on its safety or effectiveness for those suffering from RA and it may indeed interact with medications.

Green-lipped Mussel Extract

There is no reliable evidence to support the use of green-lipped muscle extract to alleviate OA or RA.

Chapter Two
Osteoarthritis (OA)

OA is a common disease, typically affecting the hips, knees and small joints in the hands, but any joint can be affected. Severity of the disease can vary and affects each person differently.

OA is a gradual loss of the cartilage which cushions the ends of bones, leaving bones unprotected from rubbing against each other. This leads to; pain, swelling and impaired movement. OA can be further exacerbated by the creation of osteophytes. Osteophytes are formed when new bone is formed underneath the worn cartilage around the edge of joints, forming outgrowths and spurs.

Historically OA has been considered part of the natural aging process. However, it is now thought to be a disease, not simply 'wear and tear' or 'nature taking its course'.

Although the triggers for the development of the disease are largely unknown and much more research is needed to understand it better, it is thought that a joint injury and genetic susceptibility plays a role. Being overweight is also a risk factor for the development of OA in later life. In addition increased risk of developing OA has been noted following trauma and inflammation in the joints.

OA is a progressive disease and rather like those who suffer RA, OA sufferers often see episodic flare ups; periods of remission and flare-ups where inflammation and pain tend to peak.

OA and it's treatment increases:	Possible reasons why:	Useful information can be found in these chapters:
The risk of being under-nourished	Pain may lead to; a small appetite tiredness, low mood and mobility problems may impact on food intake Due to adopting a 'self-help' diet	Joint and arthritic conditions and being under-nourished Fact vs Fiction section of this chapter
The risk of being overweight	Due to ability to get active	Joint and arthritic conditions and being overweight Medications
Long term health risk of developing cardiovascular disease	Due to reduced activity levels and increased risk of being overweight	Cardiovascular health
Possibility for surgery	Surgical joint replacement is an increasingly effective treatment	Eating well in hospital

Key dietary manipulations important for those suffering from OA

Nutritional therapy can help to minimise the effects of the disease, its treatment and long-term health risks. The key dietary manipulations that can help OA sufferers are:

- Being a healthy weight and well nourished. Please refer to the chapters; 'how to assess nutritional status,' relevant chapters on being overweight or under-nourished and 'a well balanced healthy diet'.
- Ensure a cardiovascular healthy diet. Please refer to the chapter 'cardiovascular health'
- Decrease cartilage damage

Decrease cartilage damage using glucosamine and chondroitin

If the maintenance and repair of cartilage could be maximized, symptoms and progression of OA are likely to be improved. This is why glucosamine and chondroitin have both been investigated for the treatment of OA. They are both elements that help to make up cartilage. More specifically glucosamine is thought to help make up cartilage and increase collagen production in cartilage and chondroitin is thought to give cartilage elasticity and helps to prevent cartilage breakdown.

Evidence shows that glucosamine (usually in a form called glucosamine sulphate) may help ease pain and stiffness in people suffering mild-moderate OA in the knees. People with more severe OA in the knees or those with OA in other joints are not likely to reap any benefits. This evidence shows that glucosamine sulphate needs to be taken in large quantities and for at least 3 months for any possible benefits to be gleaned. It seems that quantities of around 1500mg a day are needed. Although more research is needed, there does not seem to be any dangerous side effects to health of taking such high doses yet nausea and indigestion have been reported.

Glucosamine sulphate is extracted from shellfish such as crab, prawn shells and lobster, so people with allergies should avoid them.

The use of glucosamine is still poorly understood and a lot more research is need to test whether taking glucosamine sulphate does indeed have a positive effect in OA, as there seems to be a high level of 'placebo effect' whereby suffers reported improvements in pain, stiffness and function despite only taking a placebo in trials. It is thought that there are psychological elements at play.

Glucosamine is often taken in combination with chondroitin. In terms of evidence for the effectiveness of chondroitin, it is still early days. Supplements in doses of around 400–800mg a day for a minimum of 2 months has been shown to bring some benefits to OA sufferers if cartilage is not severely damaged. Again, a lot more research is needed to understand whether supplements have a placebo effect or indeed a useful physical benefit.

Omega-3 fatty acids

It is often assumed by OA sufferers that, as omega-3 fatty acids are thought to have an impact on inflammation that they will be of some benefit to their disease process. In fact, there is very little evidence that omega-3s provide significant symptomatic benefit to OA sufferers, i.e. reduce swelling, stiffness or pain. However, omega-3s are an essential part of a healthy, well-balanced diet and are a vital aspect of a cardiovascular healthy diet, so sufferers of OA will benefit in terms of including more in their diet from these perspectives. Please refer to the relevant chapter for more information.

Fact or fiction – nutrition and OA

I have met many people who have adopted 'alternative' nutritional advice from various unreliable sources. The advice from these sources was trusted, as it was presented in such a way that suggested the principles were safe and well researched.

However, these 'alternative' diets are often strict, eliminating essential food groups, and hence nutrients from the diet or add in expensive supplements that are simply of no benefit. In addition advice from these sources can be expensive. The majority of alternative diets at best do not promote health and wellbeing and at worst compromise health and wellbeing.

It is well known that nutrition has a direct impact on health. There are many different 'alternative' diets that are promoted for people suffering from OA the claims of which can sometimes be confusing. The episodic flare-ups seen in OA are easily attributed to external factors such as diet or lifestyle. This lends weight to many claims of certain faddy approaches. However, at the moment the triggers or episodic nature of OA is poorly understood.

It is absolutely understandable why the idea that simple dietary answers help fight OA, is very appealing. Claims are made that special diets, certain foods and supplements may help to cure or alleviate symptoms, but most claims are unproven and could be harmful rather than helpful. There is however, a wealth of reliable scientific evidence which shows that a healthy, well balanced diet supports the human body for good health and wellbeing. For more information on a healthy well balanced diet please refer to this chapter.

How to spot a faddy, unproven dietary claim

- Does the diet ask for the elimination of a complete food group, such as dairy?
- Does the diet ask for the elimination of a list of certain foods?
- Does the diet have any potentially harmful effects?
- Does the diet use personal testimonies, instead of scientific evidence, to support it?
- Does the diet ask for expensive supplements?

Before starting any special diet or taking any OA remedy, it is important to discuss with a qualified health professional; any evidence for effectiveness, any side-effects or possibly harmful interaction with prescription medicine.

Vitamins and mineral supplementation

Vitamin and mineral supplementation is commonly advocated to those suffering from OA. And, it may be required in some people who suffer from proven deficiencies or are undergoing certain treatments guided by a health professional. However, there is no evidence that supplementing vitamins and minerals as a routine habit, is needed or indeed has any positive effects for people with OA. In fact, simply supplementing the diet with different vitamins and minerals without the guidance of a health professional could put health at risk. This is because the different vitamins and minerals work in synergy with each other. If there is an 'overdose' of one and a lack of the other, their functions are likely to be disrupted. And, taking too much of certain vitamins or minerals (particularly the fat soluble ones) can be unhealthy, as levels can build up in the body to 'toxic' levels.

Despite some media reports or sales pitches research into supplementation with; vitamin C, vitamin E, selenium, zinc and pantothenic acid have found no proven significant benefits for those with OA.

Vitamins and minerals

These are chemicals that are needed by the body, often in small quantities, to perform essential functions. Most can not be made by the body itself, so they are an essential part of a healthy well balanced diet.

Fat soluble vitamins – Vitamin A, D, K and E

This means they are found and stored in fats within the diet and the body. It is therefore possible that stores can be built up over a lifetime, meaning that there can be large stores within the body which could potentially become excessive if consumption exceeds need.

Water soluble vitamins – Vitamins B and C

This means they are found within foods containing water and that they are needed in frequent regular intakes, as any excess intakes are excreted in the urine. Therefore risk of deficiency is high for those with a lack of variety in the diet.

Detoxification

Some claim that detoxification can help to ease OA symptoms. However, even the idea of 'detoxifying' the human body has absolutely no scientific credibility. In fact it is regarded as potentially highly dangerous to health and wellbeing. The human body regulates itself and excretes waste on a daily basis – it does not require strict detoxification and there are absolutely no benefits for those with OA.

Food allergies

There is no evidence that any kind of food allergy or intolerance has a link to the disease process of OA. Undertaking a self-imposed elimination diet in order to try and test for a food allergy or intolerance cause pose risks to health and wellbeing.

A word of warning

There are many 'food allergy' tests out there that claim to be able to diagnose from; a few drops of blood, strands of hair or a skin prick test of a range of foods for example.

Being able to identify a true food allergy (and hence the only way to be able to find out what is going on, to be able to make the most effective changes to the diet) takes close and careful monitoring. Don't get fooled. The process of identifying a true food allergy is an extensive process that needs to be undertaken with a qualified health professional. If anybody claims otherwise, it's likely that they are trying to con people out of money. And, the consequences of listening to these 'experts in food allergy' may actually negatively affect health. Always seek advice form a qualified health professional.

Dairy products

It is a common myth that dairy products cause and exacerbate OA. However, there is no good quality scientific evidence to support this theory.

CMO

CMO (otherwise known as cetyl myristoleate) is derived from beef tallow and is often promoted as a cure for OA and RA. However, there is no good quality scientific evidence to support its use. In fact it is potentially very dangerous, as people are advised to stop taking their regular arthritis medications with on CMO.

MSM

MSM (otherwise known as methyl sulfonyl methane) is also claimed to be a 'cure' all for OA and RA. However, there is no good quality scientific evidence to support its use.

Acidity regulation

It is a common myth that cutting out foods that are themselves acidic, such as acidic fruits; grapefruit, lemons and oranges will reduce the symptoms of OA. However, there is no good quality scientific evidence to support this theory.

Apple cider vinegar and honey

The use of cider vinegar follows a long tradition, having been used as a medicine for centuries. Some people believe that OA is caused by the build up of acid in the body, which crystallizes and lodges between the joints. These crystals then become surrounded by fluids, causing swelling, soreness and stiffness.

It would seem clear therefore, that cutting down on acid entering the body and foods that increase acidity within the body, may help reduce OA symptoms and progression. It is claimed that by adding cider vinegar and honey into the diet in large quantities is alkalising. However – apart from simply anecdotal claims, there is no good quality scientific evidence to support this theory or practice. Much more research is needed to investigate the safety and effectiveness of this approach.

No evidence has found benefits for OA sufferers by taking cider vinegar and honey.

Oils

It is thought that some oils, such as evening primrose, hemp, blackcurrant seed and borage seed (rich in a type of fatty acid called GLA) may benefit people with OA and RA, as GLA is said to have anti-inflammatory properties. GLA is an essential fatty acid (EFA) in the omega-6 family, found primarily in plant-based oils. For more information on omega-6 and omega-3 oils, please refer to the 'omage-3 fatty acid' chapter.

Initial studies have looked at supplementing high dose GLA (at around 1.4g /day) for at least 6 months and found it may help to reduce pain and joint swelling. However, it is still early days and more research is needed to understand the ideal dose of GLA and whether it has any safety issues supplementing at these high doses. For example it is known that GLA may increase the possibility of miscarriage.

Studies that have looked specifically at Evening Primrose Oil (EPO) have shown that they may help to relieve inflammation. EPO needs to be taken as a minimum of 3–6 months before positive effects can be seen. And, EPO needs to be taken continuously in order for the benefit to continue.

Spirulina otherwise known as Blue-Green algae, is rich in proteins, vitamins, minerals and GLA. It is thought that spirulina may help to reduce inflammation. Supplements like this derived from seaweed, have been claimed to help improve pain and stiffness. But, because of the potential for side effects and interactions with medications, supplements should be taken only under the supervision of a qualified health professional and should not be taken during pregnancy because they may be harmful. At the moment the research is still sparse and not sufficient to be able to provide advice on the safety or effectiveness or algae derived supplements.

Olive oil is also known to possess anti-inflammatory properties, but again more research is needed to understand it's potential impact on OA and RA. It would seem prudent to switch from using spreads that are made from vegetable oils or using vegetable oils in cooking, to use olive oil and olive oil based spreads.

> **There is no evidence that supplementing the diet with certain vitamins or minerals, herbal remedies, cider vinegar or honey will bring significant symptomatic or health benefits to those suffering OA.**

Herbal remedies

Despite sales claims, there is very little scientific evidence that herbal remedies help alleviate symptoms of OA. In fact, there is very little scientific evidence to support the safety of taking herbal remedies. More research is needed to understand how these herbal remedies react with common OA medications (as they could affect efficacy and may have toxic effects) and whether these herbal remedies are safe to take at all.

Chapter Three
Gout

Gout can be an extremely painful condition, thought to be caused by high levels of uric acid in the body.

Substances called purines, found in the diet and produced by the body as a natural part of living processes, are broken down in the body into uric acids. Uric acids (urate) are a waste product, which is normally passed out in the urine.

- High uric acid levels in the bloodstream = urate crystals can be deposited in joints = the joints become inflamed causing pain and discomfort
- High uric acid levels in the bloodstream = urate crystals can be deposited in cartilage = causing pain and discomfort

Uric acid levels in the bloodstream are often high in people suffering gout. High uric acid levels, also called hyperuricamia, can be caused by a decreased ability to excrete purines or an overproduction of them by the body.

Gout sufferers usually experience a sudden onset of pain and discomfort in the joint of the big toe, although it can affect any other joint. Symptoms include; inflammation and swelling of the joint and red, shiny or flaky itchy skin over the joint.

If left untreated, gout can develop into a progressive condition, with increasing damage and pain in joints and cartilage, often affecting mobility and quality of life.

However if treated, joints will usually reduce in pain and inflammation and in most sufferers, can return to normal after 3–10 days. The sooner sufferers are treated, the more quickly they will recover and the pain and discomfort will pass.

It is not known exactly what causes gout. Some people with raised uric acid levels never go on to develop it and some people with normal uric acid levels develop it. It is thought that it is a combination of factors that increase the risk of developing the condition.

The risk factors for developing gout are; being male, having excessive intakes of purine rich foods, some medications, being overweight, suffering from certain conditions including; high blood pressure, high cholesterol levels, cardiovascular disease, diabetes, poor kidney function and psoriasis. It is likely that there is also a genetic component to being at risk of developing gout, with 20% of sufferers having a close relative with the condition; their body simply either produces too much uric acid or does not eliminate it properly.

Steroid treatment is usually the first line for those suffering gout, helping to reduce inflammation initially. Then, longer-term medication is needed to either reduce the production of purines or to increase uric acid excretion. Before these medications were developed, dietary manipulation of purines was the main focus of the treatment. However, nowadays medications are effective forms of treatment in gout and therefore dietary manipulation is usually not the focus. There are some cases where engaging with dietary manipulation can be useful, for example in those who are unable to take certain medications or for gout in it's early stages.

Key dietary manipulations important for those suffering from gout

Nutritional therapy can help to minimise the effects of the disease and help in its prevention and treatment. The key dietary manipulations that can help gout sufferers are:

* Being a healthy weight
* Ensuring a cardiovascular healthy diet
* Sticking within healthy alcohol drinking guidance
* Drinking plenty of fluids
* Adapting the purine content of the diet

Sticking within healthy alcohol drinking guidance

Drinking excessive alcohol is associated with gout. This is thought to be because drinking excessively is associated with weight gain, which impacts directly on uric acid levels, or because some types of alcohol have high purine contents. Whichever the cause, it is recommended to try and stick within the healthy guidelines for drinking alcohol.

Alcohol contains 'empty calories' in that it is high in calories without providing many nutrients for good health. Drinking may also contribute to weight gain in terms of its affect on eating behaviours. Studies show that drinking alcohol in excess may lead to overeating, as it can affect judgement and contribute to eating more than might have been intended. Drinking alcohol can also increase the likelihood that weight gain is stored around the waist rather than the hips, which is associated with more negative health impacts.

Drinking too much alcohol can also lead to a wide range of health problems, including cancer, liver disease, stroke, high blood pressure and can affect mental health.

Health experts recommend that women drink no more that 2–3 units of alcohol a day and men no more than 3–4 units a day. Alcohol is broken down in the liver. Women have smaller livers than men, so tend to be affected by alcohol more quickly. Alcohol also tends to stay in their bodies for longer. That's why the recommended limit of alcohol for women is less than that for men.

A unit is half a pint of standard strength beer, lager or cider or one pub measure of spirits (25ml). A small (125ml) glass of wine is about 11/2 units. Units increase with the strength of the drink, so a stronger strength beer or wine will contain more units.

Top tips to reduce alcohol intake

✓ Some drinks now contain their unit measures on the bottle – read them and take note of the contents.
✓ Try to be aware of the unit measure in favourite tipples.
✓ Keep a diary of alcohol drinking habits – this may help to keep track and notice patterns.

✓ Match every alcoholic drink with a non-alcoholic one, such as water or low calorie soft drinks.

✓ Dilute drinks such as wine with soda water or lemonade and ice to make them last longer.

✓ Watch the size of the glass, there will be a big difference in unit measures between a 125ml glass of wine and a 250ml glass.

✓ Plan alcohol free days. If tempted to drink when out socialising, try to plan events that mean it's easier to avoid the bar such as a country walk, the cinema or a picnic.

Drinking plenty of fluids

High levels of uric acid may increase the risk of it crystallizing in the urine. It is therefore recommended to increase fluid consumption to help reduce this risk. Consult with a qualified health professional who will be able to provide personalised guidance on the amount of fluid recommended to reduce this risk and the recommend composition of fluids. Some people may need to increase intake to around 3 litres a day.

Adapt the purine content of the diet

Contrary to some beliefs, the impact that adapting purines in the diet has on uric acid levels in the body is very small. For most people suffering gout, adapting purines will make little impact on their condition. It is recommended however, to avoid *excessive* intakes of purine rich foods. This may help to avoid exacerbation of the condition and/or prevention of recurrence. Total avoidance of these foods is not usually recommended, but regular consumption may be.

Purine rich foods

- Yeast and yeast extracts
- Beer, stout and port
- Some vegetables; spinach, beans, lentils, peas, cauliflower, asparagus, mushrooms
- Meat extracts
- Some meats; kidney, heart, sweetbreads, liver, veal, turkey
- Some fish; sprats, mackerel, sardines, shrimps, whitebait, herring, fish roes, crab, anchovies, scallops, mussels

---

Fact or fiction – nutrition and gout

Before starting any special diet or taking any gout remedy, it is important to discuss with a qualified health professional; any evidence for effectiveness, any side-effects or possible harmful interaction with prescription medicine.

Adapting the diet can cure gout

The evidence shows that the impact adapting the diet can have on uric acid levels in the body is very small. The main focus of treatment is medication. Prevention of further attacks can be supported by healthy living and avoiding excessive intakes of purine rich foods.

Herbal remedies can cure gout

Despite sales claims, there is very little scientific evidence that herbal remedies help alleviate symptoms of gout. In fact, there is very little scientific evidence to support the safety of taking herbal remedies full stop

Remedies that claim to boost the blood's cleaning power for uric acid

The liver and kidneys work to clear the bloodstream of waste products, like uric acid. In some cases if these organs are not functioning effectively, uric acid levels can be affected. However, using remedies that claim to boost the body's ability to cleanse blood are potentially dangerous. Always consult a qualified health professional before considering taking anything of this kind. Many remedies lack evidence of safety and effectiveness to support their claims.

Drinking black cherry juice

Black cherry juice, available as a juice or as an extract in tablet form, has been claimed to prevent gout attacks and shorten the length of attacks. There are no robust scientific studies to support its use for gout prevention or treatment.

Part Two
Useful Chapters to Pick and Choose

Chapter Four

How to Measure Nutritional Status

How to measure nutritional status

There are a number of ways to measure nutritional status which look at different aspects of the body like dimensions, composition and function. Some measurements can be easily done at home, whilst others need to be done together with a health professional.

Measuring and monitoring nutritional status can provide important details to inform and guide joint and arthritic condition treatments and nutritional therapy. For those who need it, a registered dietitian can undertake individual full nutritional assessments and ongoing monitoring alongside treatment.

Measuring nutritional status at home

In order to measure and monitor nutritional status at home, a few simple assessments can be done. Both *objective* and *subjective* assessment can be useful.

Objective measurements of nutritional status

Body Mass Index

Body Mass Index (BMI) is based on a person's height and weight. It is used to provide a broad indicator of nutritional status. BMI only looks at weight and height – it is unable to actually distinguish body composition, i.e. what proportions of the body are fat, or muscle, so may not be an accurate representation of nutritional status in people who have suffered muscle loss or indeed those who have high levels of muscle mass such as bodybuilders and athletes.

$$BMI = \frac{\text{Weight (kg)}}{\text{Height}^2 \text{ (m)}}$$

> **BMI <17**   = **Seriously underweight**
> **BMI 17–20** = **Underweight**
> **BMI 20–25** = **Healthy weight**
> **BMI 26–30** = **Overweight**
> **BMI >30**   = **Very overweight**

For example if a person is 50kg and 1.7m.

$$BMI = \frac{50\text{kg}}{2.89} = 17.3 \text{ kg/m}^2 = \text{Underweight}$$

Percentage weight loss

If someone has lost weight – a useful indication of their nutritional status is not looking simply at the *amount* of weight that has been lost, but the percentage of total body weight lost over a certain period. If weight is lost quickly, then this is of greater concern than a slow steady weight loss rate.

% Weight Loss =

$$\frac{\text{Usual weight (kg)} - \text{Current Weight (kg)}}{\text{Usual Weight (kg)}} \times 100$$

For example if a person's usual weight is 60kg and 6 months later is 50kg:

$$\% \text{ Weight Loss} = \frac{60 - 50}{60} \times 100 = 16.6\%$$

> **If weight loss is less than 5% = This is not considered a significant amount of weight loss unless it is likely to be ongoing.**
>
> **If weight loss is 10–20% = This is considered a significant amount of weight loss. Working together with a registered dietitian, nutritional therapy aimed at preventing further weight loss and/or encourage weight gain, should certainly be engaged with or increased.**
>
> **If weight loss is greater than 20% = This is considered severe weight loss. Working together with a registered dietitian, nutritional therapy aimed to prevent further weight loss and/or encourage weight gain, should certainly be engaged with or increased.**

In reality, small amounts of weight loss can be easy to miss. A 5% weight loss in a 50kg person is only a loss of just 2.5 kg.

Monitoring of weight and other measurements of nutritional status helps to ensure changes are picked up quickly.

Waist circumference

Where excess fat is stored within the body, this is a reliable indicator of increased risk of developing health conditions such as cardiovascular disease, raised cholesterol, high blood pressure and diabetes. Most people have one of two body shapes; often referred to as 'apple' and 'pear' shapes. Those who fat is stored around their middle (abdomen) have an 'apple' shaped figure and tend to have greater risk of developing ill health than those whose fat is stored around their hips and thighs known as 'pear' shaped figures. To measure waist circumference:

- Find the top of the ribs and bottom of the hip bone
- Breathe out naturally whilst standing
- Place the tape measure in the middle of these points and wrap it around the waist (for many people this is where the tummy button is)
- Make a note of the measurement

	Healthy	**Increased health risk**	**High health risk**
Men	< 94cm (37")	> 94cm (37")	> 102cm (40")
Women	< 80cm (32")	> 80cm (32")	> 88cm (35")

Subjective measurements of nutritional status

Subjective measurements are just as important in the assessment of nutritional status as objective measurements. Subjective measurements can help to identify and understand specific nutritional problems and help to provide direction for appropriate nutritional therapy. If objective measurements, such as weight are unattainable the following questions can help to provide information on nutritional status.

- Have you unintentionally lost/gained weight?
- Do you feel that your clothes are looser/tighter?
- How long have your clothes felt different for?
- Have you had to adjust the tightness of your belt or watch strap recently? If so, how many notches have you adjusted by?
- Do you feel that you have experienced muscle wasting?
- Do you feel that you have experienced a reduction in fat stores?
- Do you feel that you currently retaining fluid? If so, where?
- Do you feel that your skins, nails or hair have changed in strength or health?

It can be useful to regularly document answers to the following questions, to help monitor changes in nutritional status.

Eating patterns

- Have you experiencing any changes in your usual dietary intake? If so, how long have you been experiencing them?
- What percentage of your usual dietary intake are you managing to eat at the moment?

- Do you have any persistent symptoms that are affecting your food intake? Outline these symptoms and how they affect your intake.

Activity

- Has your ability to carry out activities of everyday life changed? If so, how?
- Has your ability to provide and prepare food changed? If so, how?

Measuring nutritional status with a health professional

Nutritional status screening

Every health centre should have a nutritional status-screening tool, which is undertaken at a first outpatient appointment and on every hospital admission. A number of nutrition screening tools are used within health centres that take into consideration factors such as; diagnosis, weight changes, appetite changes and ability to eat. It can be useful to become familiar with the local nutrition-screening tool and ensure that it has been completed accurately and followed up appropriately.

The main aim of these types of tools is to identify over and under nutrition. For those people suffering joint and arthritic conditions, more detailed nutritional status assessment may be needed including; screening for certain vitamin and mineral deficiencies, investigating bone density and cardiovascular risk.

Biochemical tests of nutritional status

Using biochemical tests (from urine or blood samples) alone to determine nutritional status is not very reliable and hence not very useful. Many non-nutritional factors can influence biochemical results, making their accuracy low. Biochemical tests can be useful however, when used together with other measurements, to provide a broad picture of nutritional status and changes over a period of time.

Blood tests for vitamin and minerals

A number of biochemical tests can be carried out to determine vitamin and mineral levels in the blood and urine. Together with examination of physical symptoms and an accurate dietary history analysis, risk of any deficiencies can be assessed and treated accordingly.

Changes in body composition

Due to a reduction in activity levels commonly caused by joint and arthritic conditions and as a common consequence of the disease process in RA, changes in body composition can occur. In other words levels of body proteins and fat stores can change. It is beneficial to have measurements to assess changes in body composition undertaken regularly, to help provide accurate monitoring of nutritional status and guide appropriate and sufficient treatment and nutritional therapy. To interpret the measurements from these techniques, there are standard reference range charts that a health professional will use.

Measurements to assess changes in body composition

Overall body composition: BIA
Fat stores: Tricep Skin Fold Thickness (TSF)
Levels of body proteins: Grip strength and/or Mid arm
Muscle Circumference (MAMC)

Bioelectrical impedance analysis (BIA)

Bioelectrical impedance analysis (BIA) uses a machine which can accurately determine the composition of the body.

Figure of body composition

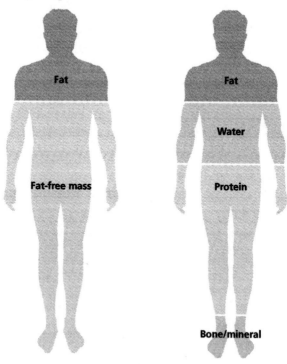

A single BIA measurement can show an individual's current body composition, which health professionals can compare with an 'ideal'. If sequential BIA measurements are taken, changes in body composition over a period of time can be tracked – which can be very useful.

Tricep skin fold thickness (TSF)

A skin fold calliper is used to measure the thickness of the tricep area to indicate body fat stores.

Grip strength

Grip strength is a functional measurement of nutritional status. A device called a handgrip dynamometer is used to test the strength of the non-dominant hand's grip. This indicates levels of muscle strength and hence levels of body proteins.

If an individual is under-nourished, functional strength is known to improve much more quickly following improvements in nutritional status compared with any other measurement. This provides a really useful early sign of improvement, which can be a great motivator; to see the response from the body to efforts of treatment and/or nutritional therapy.

Mid arm muscle circumference (MAMC)

Measurements of the circumference of the non-dominant arm, together with measurements of TSF provide an indication of muscle mass and hence levels of body proteins.

Investigating bone density

Those at risk of developing osteoporosis may be offered regular checks on their bone density. The machine used to measure bone density is called a DEXA scanner – dual energy x-ray absorptiometry.

For more information about maintaining bone health please refer to the chapter on medications.

A DEXA scanner uses low energy x-rays, through the bones. As bone blocks some of these x-rays, the denser the bones the fewer x-rays will get through to the other side. The amount of x-rays that get to the other side are measured and a computer calculates a score of the average density of the bones. A high score shows that the bone is dense and a low score that the bone is less dense and may be at risk of fracture.

Tests to assess cardiovascular health

In order to gain a better understanding of cardiovascular health and risk of cardiovascular disease, a health professional may carry out a 'cardiovascular risk assessment', which gives them an idea of the future risk of developing problems and how to direct their advice or treatment if necessary. This risk assessment involves:

- Talking about lifestyle; activity levels and smoking habits
- Learning about any family history of disease, in particular cardiovascular disease
- Testing for blood cholesterol levels by taking a small blood sample and may include taking blood sugar (glucose) levels too

- Measuring blood pressure
- Taking height, waist and weight measurements

Tests useful for those who are under-nourished

Blood tests for proteins

Certain proteins can be found in the blood stream and can give some information on nutritional status, as under-nutrition causes levels of these proteins to drop. However, these are not very reliable as there are other non-nutritional factors which can also make these protein levels to drop such as; stress, fluid balance changes within the body, administration of blood products and disease processes themselves.

Nitrogen balance

When protein is broken down and used, it is broken down into its small building blocks, called amino acids. One of the major components of amino acids is nitrogen. If there is sufficient protein in the diet the body will use what it needs and then get rid of what it doesn't in the urine and usefully, nitrogen levels can be then be detected. Measuring nitrogen balance (nitrogen in – nitrogen out) is one way of learning how the body is breaking down and using proteins from the diet and the body.

Nitrogen balance can be a useful indicator of whether an individual is consuming sufficient protein. It can also be an indicator of disease status – for example those with RA and whether they are hypermetabolic and using body proteins for energy.

In order to measure nitrogen balance, dietary protein intake is monitored and urine is collected over a 24 hours period, which can then be analysed.

If more nitrogen is found to be in the urine than is eaten, this is known as a 'positive nitrogen balance'. This shows that there is more nitrogen around, hence protein, than the body actually needs, indicating that enough protein is being eaten to cover current protein requirements. If less nitrogen is found to be in the urine than is eaten, this is known as a 'negative nitrogen balance'. The body needs more nitrogen, hence a protein, than it is actually getting, showing that body proteins are probably being broken down to provide the deficit – therefore nutritional status is likely to be affected. Some people with RA may suffer from a 'negative nitrogen balance' despite consuming sufficient protein due to the disease processes associated with metabolic changes.

Chapter Five

Joint and Arthritic Conditions and Being Overweight

Being overweight has significant negative impacts on joint and arthritic conditions. Being overweight also significantly increases the risk of cardiovascular disease. For more information on cardiovascular health please refer to this chapter.

Being overweight can lead to increased impact on joints and hence reduces mobility. It is thought that every step taken increases load on the knee and hip joint by 3–5 times body weight. This is why being overweight has such a significant impact on joints.

OA generally affects weight-bearing joints so being overweight can exacerbate symptoms and the progression of the disease. Overweight RA sufferers are at risk of increased pain and discomfort in joints affected. For those suffering gout, it is known that being overweight increases uric acid levels whilst losing weight helps to significantly reduce them.

Even a modest weight loss of 5–10% of starting body weight could help to ease strain on weight-bearing joints, improve short and long term symptoms of OA and RA, treat and prevent gout and is known to have a significantly positive impact on cardiovascular health. If a modest weight loss is not achievable, then prevention of further weight gains can be a positive goal.

To lose weight, it may be useful to seek support from a registered dietitian, support group or slimming club.

There is more and more evidence out there about what are the most successful strategies to lose weight and keep it off for good. Evidence suggests that people who are the most successful at losing weight share the following key strategies:

- Eat a diet that is generally low in fat
- Eat breakfast almost every day
- Eat regular meals
- Be as active in their day-to-day lives as possible (about 60 minutes of moderate activity such as brisk walking)
- Have a 'flexible' approach to food. This means not having an 'all or nothing' approach to eating healthily, yet being able to have an occasional treat
- Limit fast food
- Keep check of their weight regularly (once a week) to catch any small slips in weight, before they can turn into bigger weight regains
- Monitor what they eat
- Stick to the same regular meal pattern at weekends as during the week
- Continue to eat healthy and be active when on holiday

The most effective way to lose weight is by focusing on having a healthy, balanced diet and if able, increasing physical activity levels.

Chapter Six

Joint and Arthritic Conditions and Being Under-nourished

The physical effects of under-nutrition, namely weight loss, are often easy to recognise. However, under-nutrition can affect all body cells, organs and functions and can have an impact on social and psychological health too.

Being well nourished can help a person to;

- Cope with the side effects of joint or arthritic treatment
- Recover and heal from treatment or surgery, with shorter hospital stays
- Fight off infections
- Feel strong
- Maintain energy levels

When the body is under-nourished all body functions can be affected.

An inadequate intake of nutrients, not only means an inadequate intake of energy, but also means a lack of essential vitamins and minerals. And hence, the effects of under-nutrition can be wide ranging.

The effect of under-nutrition on body functions

The body is made up of billions of body cells that maintain life and growth. Body cells are produced, perform a function and then die. Some body cells tend to live, performing their function, for longer than others.

Body cells that only live for a short period of time (i.e. are produced, perform a function and then die relatively quickly) are known as 'rapid turnover' cells. These cells can be seriously affected by under- nutrition because constant supplies of nutrients are needed to produce them. Therefore the functions of the body that uses these rapid turnover cells can also be seriously affected by under-nutrition. Functions of the body, which use rapid turnover cells include:

1. Digestion
2. Blood cell production
3. Immunity
4. Healing

1. Digestion

The lining of the digestive system, called the epithelium, absorbs nutrients from food and protects the body from infection. The epithelium acts as a gateway, letting nutrients in and working to keep infections out. In order to develop an infection, from bacteria or viruses, they must first gain access to the body. This could be, for example, through cuts or grazes or though the digestive system. So if the epithelium (the body's gateway) is not working efficiently, the body can become at risk of infection.

If the cells that make up the epithelium are not supplied with sufficient nutrients, the epithelium can become weak and inefficient: the bodies' ability to effectively absorb the nutrients from food is reduced and the risk of becoming under-nourished is increased.

2. Blood cell production

Under-nutrition can reduce the production of blood cells. Having a lack of red blood cells (called anaemia) reduces the bodies' capability to carry oxygen from the lungs and around the body, which can lead to tiredness and shortness of breath. Without a constant fresh supply of oxygen, body cells become unable to function, so all body functions can be affected.

3. Immunity

The body cells that work to protect the body from infection can be significantly affected by under-nutrition, which can lead to an increased risk of infections. The immune system protects the body from infection in two different ways:

A. Protection against infections entering the body (protection and defence immunity)
B. Protection from infections which have already entered the body (immune cell immunity)

The skin and the lining of the digestive system provide protection and defence immunity. Under-nutrition reduces this type of immunity by affecting these defence systems. A lack of nutrients can cause skin to become weaker, breaking more easily, and failing to protect infections from entering the body. The lining of the digestive system (the epithelium) becomes weak without a constant supply of nutrients, increasing the likelihood of infections entering the body. Under-nutrition directly affects the cells of the immune system, leading to a reduction in their number and strength.

4. Healing

The bodies' ability to heal itself can be affected by under-nutrition. Wounds find it difficult to heal, as the extra nutrients needed to rebuild body cells are in short supply.

The social and psychological effects of under-nutrition

Under-nutrition can have effects on social and psychological health too. Being under-nourished is associated with:

- A reduced ability to concentrate
- A lack of initiative
- Feelings of apathy and low mood
- Irritability

Being under-nourished can be a major concern to a person with joint or arthritic conditions and for their loved ones around them. Weight loss and associated changes in appearance can affect a person's self-image and confidence and can be a constant daily reminder of illness. A loss of appetite, classically associated with being unwell, can have a negative impact of the quality of a person's social life, as often eating and drinking plays a part. And a lack of energy can affect the ability to carry out daily activities, like shopping and cleaning which may have an impact on independence.

In addition to engaging with nutritional therapy, sometimes simply being aware of how under-nutrition can affect social and psychological spheres and acknowledging them as an aspect of the condition and its treatment, rather than being anything intentional, can help to individuals and those around them, deal with them.

A good nutritional status can help:

✓ To be able to handle joint and arthritic treatment
✓ The body to recover and heal
✓ The body to be stronger, with more energy to undertake activities of everyday life
✓ To maintain independence
✓ To be more confident
✓ To be able to ward off feelings of apathy and low mood
✓ To promote a robust immune system
✓ To maintain concentration levels

Nutritional therapy for under-nutrition

It can be common for those with joint and arthritic conditions to have a small appetite and reduced energy levels to shop and prepare foods. This may have an impact on nutritional status and wellbeing. However, using some simple techniques and tips can help to overcome these issues to optimise the diet.

The level of nutritional therapy needed will be different for everyone and may fluctuate. Some of the techniques discussed within this chapter may not be appropriate for everyone. **Always** consult a registered dietitian or qualified health professional before engaging with any kind of nutritional therapy and again if problems persists.

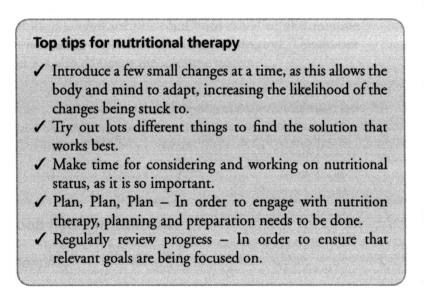

Top tips for nutritional therapy

✓ Introduce a few small changes at a time, as this allows the body and mind to adapt, increasing the likelihood of the changes being stuck to.

✓ Try out lots different things to find the solution that works best.

✓ Make time for considering and working on nutritional status, as it is so important.

✓ Plan, Plan, Plan – In order to engage with nutrition therapy, planning and preparation needs to be done.

✓ Regularly review progress – In order to ensure that relevant goals are being focused on.

A small appetite

Loss of appetite may sometimes be called anorexia. Appetite is created by and controlled through complex processes in the body. The environment and how a person thinks and feels can also influence appetite.

Providing nourishment is often naturally felt to be a way of showing care and affection: the 'food as love syndrome'. As loved ones often want to show affection for someone when they are unwell, food can sometimes become a contentious issue. Someone who has lost their appetite may feel under pressure to avoid disappointing those who have made the effort to prepare a meal for them. Meal times can cause worry and friction, taking the pleasure out of eating all together.

The key to easing friction over food is to not associate food with personal feelings and to try and share an understanding; talking about issues surrounding eating is vital. It may be easier to talk about these issues during a consultation with a registered dietitian or a support worker.

Eating is not just an adjunct to life, such as taking medicines or undergoing treatment, but is an integral part of everyday life. Eating habits evolve over a lifetime and often become deeply ingrained. Having to change these habits can often be really difficult and have a big impact on life, just like changing any other habit that has become deeply ingrained, such as giving up smoking. Acknowledging that making changes to eating can, in itself, cause anxiety could help to start easing tensions.

Food shopping, preparation, and mealtimes may need to be adapted so planning ahead is important. Learning about and being aware of how dietary intake is affected by a joint or arthritic condition, for example by a small appetite, can really help to 'set the scene' for how food can fit it more comfortably.

Some people affected by joint and arthritic conditions may have difficulties in shopping and preparing meals so may need some additional support or assistance. It may be useful to get a referral to an occupational therapist for advice on relevant local support networks and equipment available or modifications around the house that can help make life a little easier.

There are different local support networks that could offer help with shopping for and preparing food. Adaptations to everyday equipment in the kitchen can help make preparing food much easier. For example there; is a range of equipments to open bottles and cans easily like swivel taps, easy grip or easy use cutlery, easy to use scissors, trolleys and a various designs of plates, dishes and trays that can all make preparing food and eating much easier.

It may be useful to know that there are many different people that can help with problems affecting nutritional intake and support a nutritional therapy plan.

People like family and friends, support workers and specialist nurses can help to manage nutritional problems. Doctors can diagnose specific nutritional problems and advise or prescribe treatment to help overcome them. Pharmacists can help by ensuring that the type and dose of any drug prescribed is safe and they are an expert source of medication knowledge and expertise.

Registered dietitians are specifically trained in nutritional therapy and can help deal with nutritional problems. Registered dietitians undertake comprehensive nutritional assessments and monitoring and help to devise and support personalised nutritional therapy plans.

Techniques to help with a small appetite

- Try to eat 'little and often' having small meals and snacks – Instead of 3 meals a day, try to eat every 2–3 hours or have 6 small meals a day.
- Eat puddings and desserts after a break following main course.
- Friends and family could help by preparing small meals.
- Fortify the diet with additional calories and protein.
- Choose foods that appeal to the senses – for example foods that look really tasty or smell tasty.
- If the smell of food affects appetite, try to have slightly warm or cold foods.
- Have small servings of favorite foods in stock.
- Serve food in small portion – seeing and being expected to eat large portion may further reduce appetite.
- Ensure a stock of easy to make foods is in the cupboards, like soup, boil in the bag or frozen meals.
- Try to avoid drinking half an hour before and during a meal – as this may fill up the stomach with liquids, instead of nutritious food.
- Sip nutritious drinks throughout the day, like milky or sugary drinks.
- Try a small glass of alcohol half an hour before eating, as this can help to stimulate appetite.
- Try a short walk in the fresh air before eating.
- Make the table or tray look attractive with a table cloth or some flowers.
- Keep nutritious little snacks easy to hand throughout the day.
- Make the most of times when appetite is at its best, often in the mornings.

- Try eating a meal or snack in front of the television or with the radio on in the background – People naturally tend to eat more when there is some form of distraction around them.

Sample menu using techniques to help with a small appetite:

Breakfast	A small bowl of cereal with fortified whole milk and honey
	1 piece of toast with thickly spread peanut butter and a small banana
	A cup of tea made with fortified whole milk and 2 sugars
Mid morning	A small milky coffee made from fortified whole milk
	A small pot of full fat fromias frais with a handful of dried fruit sprinkled over the top
Lunch	Take a stroll in the fresh air or get out into the garden
	A small tin of creamy soup with a tablespoon of cream mixed in and grated cheese on top and a hard boiled egg

Mid afternoon	A cup of warmed fortified whole milk with 2 chocolate biscuits
Dinner	Have a small glass of favorite wine half an hour before dinner is served.
	One small sausage and 1 scoop of mash fortified with cream and grated cheese, and a tablespoon of vegetables with butter melted on the top – garnished with some fresh herbs.
	A small bowl of fruit and ice cream
Evening snack	A small slice of cake and a handful of grapes served with a cup of tea made with fortified whole milk and 2 sugars
Before bed	A small mug of malted drink made with fortified whole milk

Fortifying the nutritional content of the diet

Although a healthy, well-balanced diet is important for good health, maintaining a healthy weight and preventing becoming underweight, are often crucial goals of nutritional therapy. It is important to adapt the diet to achieve these goals, even if it means eating foods that are high in fat or sugar.

Preventing or treating under-nutrition is likely to have more beneficial effects than any negative effects from eating high fat and sugary foods. However, it is important that if sugary foods are eaten frequently that the teeth are cleaned regularly.

Food fortification can really make a difference to the overall nutritional content of the diet. For example simply switching from having semi-skimmed milk to whole milk will add 120 calories per pint. If this whole milk is then fortified with 4 tablespoons of milk powder, this will add an extra 125 calories and 13 grams of protein. The volume of milk is still only 1 pint, but the nutritional content has been boosted by 245 calories and 13 grams of protein (almost the same amount as having another pint of semi-skimmed milk).

> **Food fortification can be an easy way to add extra nutrition into everyday food, without increasing the volume, which is useful for those with a small appetite.**

How to fortify the nutritional content of everyday foods:

- If boosting the nutritional content of everyday foods is needed, then choosing full fat, high calorie options will make a good start.
- Increase the use of full fat dairy products like milk, cream, cheese and butter.
- Increase the use of sugary foods.
- Grate cheese into dishes such as soup, mashed potato or omelettes.
- Add bean, lentils or noodles into soups.
- Add double cream into soup, mashed potato and sauces or desserts.

- Add full fat milk into dishes such as mash potato or custard.
- Add evaporated milk to milk-based desserts.
- Add butter onto vegetables, pasta and potatoes.
- Add syrup or honey to breakfast cereals or desserts.
- Add sugar to foods and drinks.
- Use plenty of butter in sandwiches or on toast
- Fortify milk – Add 4 tablespoons of milk powder to one pint of whole milk. Mix well. Store in the fridge and use within 24 hours.
- Keep high calorie snacks to hand – such as nuts, cheese and biscuits, biscuits, full fat yoghurts and fromage frais.
- Add ice cream to puddings or smoothies.
- Try to make fluids as nourishing as possible – choose milky drinks or smoothies to supply fluids and nutrition. Try liquidising fresh fruit with milk, yoghurt, ice cream, or fruit juice.

Nutritional supplements

There are many different types of nutritional supplements available. Some are available to purchase in supermarkets or local pharmacies and some are only available on prescription. It can be useful to be aware of the different types available.

Some supplements can be used within recipes to help increase their uses. There may be suggestions on the back of packets or a website or a telephone number to call for further information where recipes and ideas can be requested often free of charge.

Over the counter nutritional supplements

Powders that can be made into drinks or soups and ready made drinks are available without a prescription. They can be high in calories and protein and are sometimes fortified with vitamins and minerals. These can be useful to boost the nutritional content of the diet by being used in-between meals, or they can be used to replace a meal or snack if it is not able to be eaten. It is advisable however to consult with a qualified health professional if these types of drinks are being used to replace meals, as supplements that are nutritionally complete would be more beneficial in this instance.

Nutritionally complete supplements

This type of supplement provides all the nutrition the body needs within a certain volume (i.e. energy, protein and vitamins and minerals). Nutritionally complete supplements are only available on prescription, so they can be safely prescribed and monitored. There are many different types available and a number of different companies that produce them.

There are:

- Milkshake style drinks
- Fruit juice style drinks
- Yoghurt style drinks
- Puddings
- Soups

These types of supplements should ideally be used in addition to eating and drinking. However, in some instances they may need to be used as a sole source of nutrition. Some people may dislike one brand, type or flavour but then really enjoy another. It is really important to trial as many different flavours, types and brands as possible to find the ones that are most preferable. Some companies produce 'starter packs' that contain their whole range to trial.

Techniques to get the best out of nutritional supplements

Fruit juice style drinks	Milkshake style drinks
Best served chilled	Best served chilled
Try mixing with lemonade, fresh fruit juice, fizzy water	Try mixing with some whole milk
Use in a recipes for jelly or fruit salad, trifles or fruit compote	Try adding to smoothies
Try freezing for a refreshing ice lolly or freeze as small ice cubes to suck on	Use in recipes to make rice pudding, custard, potato gratin, cakes or pancakes
Try adding to smoothies	Try adding to soups

Protein and energy supplements

Powdered supplements of protein or energy (energy in the form of sugar) are available, which can be added to everyday foods such as soups, without affecting texture or taste. In addition, there are liquid protein and energy supplements (energy in the form of fat) that can be added to everyday food or taken much like a medication. These types of supplements, often called 'modular' as they only provide one type of nutrient, are not as beneficial as nutritionally complete types, but can be useful for those who are struggling to have sufficient nutrient intakes or those that are unable to tolerate sufficient nutritionally complete supplements.

Techniques to help with tiredness

- Try out internet shopping – shopping can often be ordered and delivered free of charge.
- Ask a friend to help to put away shopping after a trip or a delivery.
- Make the most of the not so tired times, by doing the shopping or preparing meals and freezing them.
- Make the most of the array of convenience foods on the markets, such as tinned, frozen, microwave and boil-in-the-bag. Stock up on these types of meals.
- Takeaways delivered to your door can sometimes be useful.
- Ordering meals on wheels for a certain time period could be a useful option, for example over a period of a flare up or specific treatment.

Store cupboard essentials

It may be easier to eat nutritious meals, if there are nutritious, quick and easy to prepare foods in the cupboards. Try stocking up on some of the ideas below.

- Tinned beans, spaghetti, ravioli, macaroni cheese.
- Tinned fish such as tuna, salmon, mackerel. Tinned fish in sauces may make preparing a meal even easier
- Tinned soups
- Tinned fruit
- Frozen ready meals
- Boil in the bag fish
- Powdered mash potatoes
- Tinned, frozen and dried fruits
- Tinned, frozen and microwavable vegetables
- Tinned puddings
- Packet instant desserts
- Long life or powdered milk
- Crackers that are wrapped in small packs of 2–3
- Single serving packs of breakfast cereals
- Single servings of cheese
- Freshly prepared dishes like lasagna or chilli frozen in individual portions

Chapter Seven

Protect against Infection – Basic Food Hygiene

Being under-nourished and/or undergoing certain types of treatment for joint and arthritic conditions can affect the immune system – increasing the risk of catching an infection. The disease process of RA also dampens the immune system.

In these cases, it is important that any potential sources of infection are reduced as much as possible to help prevent infections. One potential source of infection comes from food and drink, so following basic food hygiene principles is sensible.

Basic food hygiene principles

Food shopping

- Avoid choosing food in damaged or broken packaging
- Avoid choosing food that is stored in overloaded fridges or freezers as they may not be cooled enough
- Try to get food shopping home as quickly as possible, and into the fridge or freezer
- Strictly observe best before or use by dates

Food storage

- Keep the freezer below −18°C.
- Keep the fridge between 0°C and 5°C
- Store cooked food at the top of the fridge and raw food at the bottom.
- Any raw meat or fish should be kept at the bottom of the fridge in covered containers
- Always store eggs in the fridge
- Never re-freeze thawed food
- Do not put hot food in the fridge, as this will increase the temperature of all food in the fridge potentially making it unsafe to eat. Cool food at room temperature within an hour after cooking and then chill or freeze

Food preparation

- Always wash hands before handling any food, in-between handling food and doing other things. Dry hands thoroughly as damp hands carry more germs.
- Dry hands using a dedicated hand drying towel or use kitchen paper – do not use a tea towel used for other uses
- Cover cuts and grazes with a waterproof plaster
- Keep pets away from the kitchen
- Disinfect work surfaces regularly
- Change or wash thoroughly anything used for raw and cooked foods, such as chopping boards, and utensils
- Wash all fruit and vegetables before eating
- Wash the top of cans before opening

Cooking food

- Always thaw frozen food in the fridge, not at room temperature
- Cook food until it is piping hot all the way through and meat until juices run clear
- Always observe the cooking instruction on the label
- Don't let raw meat touch any other foods
- Do not reheat cooked food

Eating out

- Ensure food is piping hot when served and cooked all the way through
- Choose freshly prepared foods from reputable outlets. Avoid salad bars, street vendors, market stalls and ice cream vans

Chapter Eight

Eating Well in Hospital

A common issue associated with any kind of clinical treatment can be the availability and preference of food in hospital.

Being a patient in hospital and fitting in with set meal times can be difficult. People may be asleep or resting during mealtimes, may be undergoing tests or feeling unwell. Due to food hygiene regulations, meals commonly cannot be reheated and some hospitals may only be able to provide snacks or cold foods if a hot meal is missed.

Treatment centres should always have strategies in place, so if meals are missed or people are hungry, there is food available. It can be useful to check with the centre what systems are in place and if necessary arrange and plan to take in snacks and food that are enjoyed. Check with the centre what policies are in place for bringing in food and make sure the centre is aware of any specific dietary needs or preferences. Treatment centres work to provide nutritious and enjoyable meals and snacks. However, everyone has different tastes and preferences and it can be very difficult to please everyone.

Whilst undergoing treatment, it can be difficult for people to actually eat due to tiredness, feelings of illness or being attached to drips and monitors. If this is the case, it may be useful have a little help from nurses. Having family or friends present at mealtimes can also be a great help, to choose suitable options from the menu or trolley and to offer a little help if needed.

Tips for eating well in hospital:

✓ Try to keep nutritious and tasty snacks by the bedside. Fruit is often a popular choice, but it doesn't contain much nutrition. Try and go for fruit, but also include choices such as nuts or snack bars.

✓ If well enough, plan to visit the local cafe or restaurant to have a meal of choice.

✓ Family or friends could to bring in food from home such as hot soup in a flask, a favourite sandwich or a special dessert.

✓ Family or friends could bring in a take-away.

✓ If it is possible, ask staff to put a nametag on food to be stored in the fridge such as; favourite yoghurts, milkshakes or refreshing drinks.

✓ Some treatment centres may be able to provide small fridges next to beds, to store personal food supplies and keep food and drinks chilled.

✓ Family and friends could bring in a cool box or bag to keep things cool for a while, for example refreshing drinks.

✓ Discussing needs and preferences with the member of staff who serves the food can be helpful. Staff may keep a record of these for their own reference.

✓ Discuss needs and preferences with a registered dietitian as they may be able to arrange for particular foods, meals or snacks to be provided.

✓ Family and friends could help to make sure water jugs are refreshed and filled during visits.

✓ Having a favourite squash to mix with water could help encourage fluid intake.

✓ Keeping only a small supply of snacks and treats by the bedside, but refreshing them regularly, could help to avoid boredom and food becoming stale.

✓ Eating by the bedside may not be ideal, so find out if there are allocated eating areas away from bed areas.

✓ Ensure that there is sufficient equipment to be able to eat, for example, is there a table that can reach an appropriate height and is there sufficient seating.

✓ Request to see a menu. Some hospitals do not necessarily display their menus, but they should always be available on request. Seeing the menu could help to aid choice.

✓ If the catering in hospital is not up to standard – make sure the appropriate staff are informed about the reason for dissatisfaction and any suggestions for how things may be improved. This can help improve services for the future.

Chapter Nine

A Healthy Well Balanced Diet

It is well known that nutrition has a direct impact on health. A healthy, balanced diet is vital for good health and there is no exception for people with joint or arthritic conditions.

No one single food or food group can provide the human body with all the nutrients it needs, so having a varied diet is key. However, the body does requires different nutrients in differing amounts, so it stands to reason that different food groups are needed in differing proportions.

For good health the body needs: Regular meals which are based on fibre rich starchy carbohydrates (like pasta, bread, rice, potatoes or cereals), with plenty of fruit and vegetables (at least five portions every day), some lean or low fat protein-rich foods (such as meat, fish, eggs, lentils, milk and dairy) and a small amount of healthy fats. Not forgetting plenty of fluids (6–8 glasses or around 1.2 litres a day) to keep the body hydrated.

Focus on carbohydrates

There are two types of carbohydrate: sugars and starch. The majority of the energy in the diet should come from fibre rich starchy carbohydrates like brown bread, cereals, rice, pasta and potatoes. Sugary carbohydrates, like those found in honey, chocolate, cakes, biscuits and fizzy drinks, can also provide an important source of energy, particularly if someone has a small appetite. If someone has a small appetite, then aiming for a fibre rich diet may not be appropriate as it tends to fill up the stomach without many calories. Conversely, if someone is trying to lose weight aiming for a fibre rich diet may be effective in helping to fill them up, without many calories.

Carbohydrates could help to preserve body proteins in those who are under-nourished

All body cells need a constant supply of fuel. Glucose is the main source of fuel for the body. When carbohydrates are eaten, the body breaks them down into their simplest form – glucose. But, if carbohydrates are in short supply, glucose can also be obtained by breaking down body proteins.

If there are insufficient supplies of carbohydrates for body fuel, body proteins are raided. In order to help to preserve body proteins, an adequate amount of carbohydrates is vital. As RA causes changes in carbohydrate metabolism (by reducing its efficiency), the amount of carbohydrate needed to help preserve body proteins is increased. Sugary carbohydrates found in sugary drinks, chocolate and sweets could be an excellent way to provide energy for the body when someone has a small appetite.

Focus on fruit and vegetables

A healthy diet consists of at least five portions of fruit and vegetables every day, these can be fresh, frozen, dried or tinned. Roughly, a portion of fruit and vegetables fits within the palm of the hand. Aiming to have a variety of different fruit and vegetables will help to ensure a variety of vitamins and minerals.

Achieving at least five portions may sound like rather a lot, but planning ahead and thinking about how to achieve this level by the end of day – will certainly help. Trying to include fruit and vegetables at each meal and snacks should mean that reaching the 5 a day target is easy.

Ways to achieve 5 a day:

> Breakfast: Add strawberries, raisons or dried fruit to cereal or yoghurt (1) and have a small glass of fruit juice (2).
> Mid Morning: Have a piece of fruit as a snack, such as an apple, 2 plums or a cupful of grapes (3).
> Lunch: Have salad in a sandwich or accompanying meal (4).
> Mid Afternoon: Have another piece of fruit, such as a banana or orange (5). Aim to keep it varied.
> Evening Meal: Have an vegetable packed meal serving 2–3 portions (7–8).

Focus on protein

Proteins are made up of smaller elements called amino acids. There are 20 different types of amino acids. It is these small amino acids, often called the building blocks of life that the body uses to build and repair itself. The body needs a supply of all the 20 different amino acids to work properly.

Amino acids are found in two groups:

1. Non-essential amino acids – these types of amino acids can be made within the body from the ingredients of other amino acids. There are 12 different types of non- essential amino acids.
2. Essential amino acids – these types of amino acids cannot be made within the body. The only way that the body can get some is from the diet. There are 8 different types of essential amino acids.

Different protein rich foods contain different amounts and combinations of amino acids. This is why the choice of protein rich foods is important, as it can have an impact on whether there are sufficient amino acids in the diet to make sure that the body is able to work properly.

The biological value of different protein rich foods is the measure of how sufficient it is in all the amino acids needed for the body. Foods classed as high biological value are those that are sources of all the essential amino acids needed for the body. Foods classed as low biological value are those that do not have all the essential amino acids needed for the body.

High biological value protein sources include; protein from animal sources, such as meat and dairy products, fish, eggs, beans, lentils and soya products. Low biological value protein sources include; bread, vegetables, nuts, and seeds.

How much protein do we actually need?

We have an essential need to include protein in our diets everyday. However, we don't actually need very much of it: we only need two to three portions of different protein-rich foods each day.

It is often thought that eating large amounts of protein, such as lots of eggs or high protein shakes will help build muscle mass. In fact this is not the case. If we eat more protein than our bodies need, the body cannot store it anywhere, so it simply gets rid of it.

For those people with reduced dietary intakes, choosing protein sources that are high biological value can help to prevent under nutrition.

Focus on healthy fats

Although a high fat diet is unhealthy, a healthy diet does include some 'healthy' fats. Please refer to the cardiovascular health chapter for a low down on different types of fats.

Focus on vitamin and minerals

A healthy, balanced diet should provide all the vitamins and minerals the body needs. However, treatments associated with joint and arthritic conditions mean that some people may be at risk of deficiencies.

Taking vitamin and mineral supplements unsupervised is not advisable, particularly for people with joint and arthritic conditions. This is because any deficiencies that are not properly treated could cause a problem. And taking doses of supplements that are not appropriately balanced can lead to imbalances in vitamins and minerals that can be toxic, affect health or interfere with treatment. It is advisable to discuss vitamin and mineral supplementation with a qualified health professional to ensure that any potential deficiencies can be properly identified and safely corrected.

Focus on fluids

The body needs around 6 to 8 glasses (1.2 litres) of fluid, every day. When the weather is warm or the body is active, it will need more. Ensuring a regular and sufficient fluid intake is vital. Feelings of thirst actually indicate that the body is already getting dehydrated, so drinking before getting thirsty is advisable.

Chapter Ten
Cardiovascular Health

Cardiovascular disease is a term used to describe a number of conditions involving the heart and blood vessels which can lead to heart attacks, heart failure and stroke. The best ways to keep the heart and blood vessels in healthy condition is to consume a healthy diet, increase physical activity levels and stop smoking.

Those suffering from joint and arthritic condition can be at a higher risk of developing cardiovascular disease, due to side effects of the condition, the disease process itself, decreased mobility and overweight and/or side effects of medications.

Following a healthy well balanced diet is vital to: reduce the risk of developing cardiovascular disease, maintain a healthy weight, reduce blood pressure, lower cholesterol levels and to help prevent blood clotting. An ideal cardiovascular healthy diet is one that is:

1. High in fruit and vegetables
2. Low in saturated and trans fats with sufficient omega-3s
3. Low in salt
4. Rich in whole grains
5. Includes alcohol within sensible limits

1. High in fruit and vegetables: Getting at least 5 a day has great benefits for heart and blood vessel health. This is because they are packed full of vitamins, minerals, fibre and antioxidants which help protect them. Around 30% of cardiovascular disease in the western world is thought to be directly caused by a low consumption of fruit and vegetables. It really does pay to get in 5 a day.

2. Low in saturated and trans fats, with sufficient omega-3s: High amounts of saturated and trans fats increase blood cholesterol levels which can increase the risk of developing cardiovascular disease. For more information on omega-3s, please refer to this chapter.

The low down on fats

Consult with a qualified health professional to get regular checks of blood cholesterol levels.

Saturated fat

- Found in foods such as the fat on red meat and poultry, cakes, biscuits, pastries, butter, suet, ghee, lard, full fat dairy products, tropical oils such as palm, palm kernel and coconut.
- This is the unhealthiest type of fat and should be avoided as it raises unhealthy blood cholesterol levels which increase the risk of cardiovascular disease.

Polyunsaturated fat

- Polyunsaturated fats can be found in vegetable oils such as safflower, corn, sunflower, sesame, soybean, cottonseed and walnut oils.

- This type of fat is preferred to saturated fat as it lowers unhealthy blood cholesterol levels. However, it is not as healthy as monounsaturated fats, as it can lower healthy blood cholesterol levels too.

Monounsaturated fat

- Good sources of monounsaturated fat include nuts, olives, avocados and oils such as canola, peanut and olive.
- Monounsaturated fats are the healthiest type of fat and should make up most of the fat in the diet. This type of fat helps to lower the unhealthy blood cholesterols but does not affect the healthy blood cholesterols.
- Research suggests that people who consume diets rich in monounsaturated fats have low rates of cardiovascular disease.

Trans fatty acids

- Trans fatty acids are formed during the manufacturing process that turns liquid fats into solid fats (the process called hydrogenation). This process prolongs the shelf life of foods by making them less likely to turn rancid. It also improves the texture and baking quality of foods, making pie crust flaky, margarine spreadable and puddings creamy.
- This type of fat is unhealthy because they raise unhealthy blood cholesterols and also lower healthy blood cholesterols.

Most of the trans fat in the UK diet comes from processed foods. In addition, there is a small amount of naturally occurring trans fat in several animal based foods. Avoiding processed food containing trans fats would be a healthy decision. Try to avoid hydrogenated vegetable fat oils, shortenings, cakes, biscuits, chocolate, pastry, sauces and oils used repeatedly for deep frying such as fast foods and takeaways.

Label smart

A quick way to tell if a food is high in fat is to check food labels. Look for the amount per 100g.

Foods that are **High** in fat have 20g of more of fat per 100g. Foods that are **High** in saturated fat have 5g of more of saturated fat per 100g.

Foods that are **Low** in fat have 3g or less of fat per 100g
Foods that are **Low** in saturated fat have 1.5g or less of saturated fat per 100g.

---

3. Low in salt: Having too much salt in the diet increases blood pressure, which increases the risk of developing cardiovascular disease. In fact, when blood pressure is above healthy levels people are three times more likely to develop cardiovascular disease or have a stroke compared to people with a healthy blood pressure.

The body does need salt in small amounts for a variety of functions, including:

- Nerve and muscles functions
- Regulation of body fluids
- Taking nutrients from the bloodstream into body cells

But most people in the western world are eating far too much. For good health, we should be having no more than 6 grams of salt a day, which is about one teaspoon. Many people consume around 9g per day-a third too much. Adding salt to cooking and on dishes at the table can add flavour, but it is easy to over do it, quickly adding up to much more than a teaspoon. Around 75%, of the salt we consume is 'hidden' in processed foods, so the simplest way to cut down on salt is to eat more fresh foods and to avoid adding salt at cooking and the table. Try replacing salt in dishes and cooking with: fresh or dried herbs, spices, pepper, vinegar or mustards.

Consult with a qualified health professional to get regular blood pressure level checks.

Label smart

A quick way to tell if a food is high in salt is to check food labels. Look for the amount 100g.

Foods that are **High** in salt have 1.5g of more of salt per 100g (or 0.6g sodium).

Foods that are **Low** in salt have 0.3g or less of salt per 100g (or 0.1g sodium).

4. Rich in whole grains: Whole grains are the seeds of a grain food that can be eaten as a whole. When grains are refined by modern milling techniques, the seeds are broken down and the majority of the very healthy fibre, B vitamins, vitamin E and minerals naturally found in the wholegrain are lost.

Intakes of refined grains such as white pasta, white bread and breakfast cereals are increasing. However, diets rich in whole grains are linked to decreased risks of cardiovascular disease, type 2 diabetes and some cancers. Try to choose wholegrain varieties of food choices whenever you can. Choose food that says 'wholegrain' or 'whole' before the name of the grain on the packaging or in the ingredient list.

The following are typical wholegrain products:

- Wholemeal breads
- Whole wheat pasta
- Whole grain breakfast cereals.
- Brown rice
- Wild rice
- Oats
- Popcorn
- Barley
- Bulgur wheat
- Millet
- Quinoa
- Rye
- Spelt

5. Includes alcohol within sensible limits: Moderate alcohol consumption is thought to reduce the risk of cardiovascular disease. Red wine for example, is said to have health benefits because it contains flavanoids (a type of antioxidant) that are believed to help prevent cardiovascular disease. There is evidence to suggest that having 1–2 units of alcohol a day may help protect against disease. But, this is not universally beneficial as this effect has only been shown for men over 40 and for women after the menopause.

Alcohol intakes over the healthy recommendations have been shown to increase the risk of cardiovascular disease.

Alcohol contains 'empty calories' in that it is high in calories without providing many nutrients for good health. Drinking may also contribute to weight gain in terms of its affect on eating behaviours. Studies show that drinking alcohol in excess may lead to overeating, as it can affect judgement and contribute to eating more than might have been intended. Drinking alcohol can increase the likelihood that weight gain is stored around the waist rather than the hips, which is associated with more negative health.

Drinking too much alcohol can also lead to a wide range of health problems including; cancer, liver disease, stroke, high blood pressure and can affect mental health.

Health experts recommend that women drink no more that 2–3 units of alcohol a day and men no more than 3–4 units a day. Alcohol is broken down in the liver. Women have smaller livers than men, so tend to be affected by alcohol more quickly. And, alcohol also tends to stay in their bodies for longer. That's why the recommended limit of alcohol for women is less than that for men.

A unit is half a pint of standard strength beer, lager or cider or one pub measure of spirits (25ml). A small (125ml) glass of wine is about 11/2 units. Units increase with the strength of the drink, so a stronger strength beer or wine will contain more units.

Being a healthy weight is important to reduce the risk of cardiovascular disease

Being overweight significantly increases the risk of developing cardiovascular disease, but the good news is that weight loss can help to decrease this risk. Research has shown that the likelihood of developing cardiovascular disease is about 75% greater for overweight women compared to women at a healthy weight, with risk tripling for women with a BMI higher than 29. Overweight men have a 58% increased risk of the disease and obese men having more than double the risk. Please refer to the 'joint and arthritic conditions and being overweight' chapter for more information about being overweight and tips for healthy weight loss.

Chapter Eleven

Omega-3 Fatty Acids

Omega-3 fatty acids have been shown to: reduce the risk of heart disease by lowering levels of fat in the blood, reduce the risk of blood clotting in some people, reduce the risk of hypertension and some types of cancer and may have a role in supporting the treatment of joint and arthritic conditions.

What are omega-3 fatty acids?

Omega-3 fatty acids, sometimes called omega-3s, omega-3 oils or n3s, are a type of essential fatty acid. This means that the body must get a source of it in the diet, as it cannot produce it itself (i.e. essential).

Fats are made up of smaller building blocks called fatty acids. There are 3 main types of fatty acids; saturated, unsaturated and monounsaturated. There are 2 subgroups of unsaturated fatty acids; omega-6s and omega-3s.

Omega-3 fatty acids are available in 3 different forms; alpha-linolenic acid (ALA), eicosapentanenoic acid (EPA), and docosahexaenoic acid (DHA). ALA is found mostly in plant-based foods; EPA and DHA are found mostly in oily fish.

The body is able to convert ALA to EPA and DHA, but it does not yield as much omega-3s compared with consuming EPA and DHA directly.

As part of a healthy protein intake, it is recommended to have at least two portions of fish a week (a portion is about 140g), one of which should be oily. For women of childbearing age and those pregnant or breastfeeding, they should have no more than 2 portions of oily fish a week. Women who will not have a baby in the future and men should have no more that 4 portions of oily fish a week (this is due to the possibility of building up low levels of pollutants called dioxins and PCBs in the body). The health benefits of consuming oily fish are significant.

Oily fish:

- Salmon
- Trout
- Mackerel
- Kippers
- Sardines
- Herrings
- Anchovies
- Carp
- Eel
- Pilchards
- Sprats
- Swordfish
- Fresh tuna – when tuna is canned omega-3s tend to be lost
- Whitebait

There are some suggestions that if someone does not consume oily fish that omega-3s can be provided through plant-based sources. However, research shows that the type of fatty acid in plant-based sources (ALA) may not have the same general health benefits of those in fish EPA and DHA. And, research suggests that plant based omega-3 sources are not as effective at relieving joint symptoms and arthritic conditions.

NB: Cod liver oils do not contain omega-3s. Omega-3s are found in the flesh of oily fish, so this needs to be consumed in order to glean the nutritional benefits.

Plant based sources of omega-3 fatty acids:

- Flaxseed
- Canola oil
- Soybeans
- Linseed
- Walnuts
- Tofu
- Omega-3 rich eggs (the chickens have been fed a high flaxseed diet

The omega-6:omega-3 ratio (or sometimes called n6:n3)

It is thought that omega-3s 'compete' with omega-6s to undertake natural functions in the body effectively. If there is too much omega-6s in the body, they will 'overpower' omega-3s, making them less effective.

In the Western World, consumption of omega-6 fatty acids tends to be excessive, whilst consumption of omega-3 fatty acids tends to be insufficient. It is thought this imbalance increases the risks of inflammatory disorders, heart disease and some cancers, whereas a lower ratio of omega-6s to omega-3s is thought to have a healthier, opposite effect. This is because omega-3s are anti-inflammatory and excessive intakes of omega-6s are pro-inflammatory (meaning they increase inflammation).

Adapting the diet to have less omega-6s and more omega-3s is recommended for good health and wellbeing and may help to support the management of joint and arthritic conditions.

The main sources of omega-6s in the diet include: corn and sunflower oils, margarines and processed foods made with these oils. It can easy to consume omega-6s without knowing it, as consumption of processed foods is ever increasing.

Simply reducing the amounts of processed foods and replacing cooking oils for monounsaturated based oils like olive, soybean or canola and increasing consumption of oily fish, will help to improve the ratio of fatty acids in the diet.

Chapter Twelve

Medications Commonly Used to Treat Joint and Arthritic Conditions

Some medications can increase the body's basic requirements for nutrients or decrease their absorption from food. Nutritional therapy can help to minimise the side effects of medication needed for joint and arthritic conditions. The three predominantly used medications for joint and arthritic conditions, and their nutritional implications, are discussed in this chapter. Discuss with a qualified health professional, personal prescriptions and implications.

Nonsteroidal anti-inflammatory drugs (NSAIDs)

Common NSAIDs such as aspirin or ibuprofen, work by blocking chemicals in the body called prostaglandins that help to spark inflammation. NSAIDs relieve pain, reduce inflammation and lower a high temperature.

Prostaglandins also play a role in the health of the stomach lining, which means that some users can suffer heartburn, indigestion and/or sickness and may have an increased risk of stomach or duodenal ulceration. Please refer to the end of this chapter for some advice on how to optimise eating when feeling unwell.

Prescription of medication to help protect against stomach lining ulceration and to help reduce indigestion are often given. Oral

NSAIDs should be taken with or after food or milk, as this makes it less likely that the NSAIDs will cause these stomach problems.

Corticosteriods

Corticosteroids are any type of medication that contains steroids, a type of hormone in the body. Corticosteriods can reduce inflammation and suppress the immune system. As corticosteroids are hormones, they have the potential to affect a wide range of body processes. The side effects of taking this type of medication will vary depending on the type, strength and length that it is taken for.

Corticosteroids can be inhaled, injected into muscles or joints, taken orally or injected into the bloodstream. If the medication is taken orally or in the bloodstream, it tends to have side effects throughout the body system. However taking it inhaled or injected into muscles or joints helps to keep it's effects localized.

Those with joint and arthritic conditions generally take corticosteroids orally, into muscles or joints or into the bloodstream.

Corticosteroids injected into the bloodstream can cause side effects that impact on the ability and enjoyment to eat including: indigestion and heartburn, nausea and a metallic taste in the mouth. Please refer to the end of this chapter for some advice on how to optimise eating when feeling unwell.

Corticosteroids taken orally can increase appetite and increase the risk of fluid retention, leading to weight gain. Taken long term it increases the risk of infection due to its action of dampening the body's immune system defenses. Please refer to the chapters: 'joint and arthritic condition and being overweight' and 'protect against infections – basic food hygiene'.

Oral corticosteriods have been shown to increase the body's excretion of zinc, calcium and nitrogen in the urine (therefore increasing the risk of becoming under-nourished). They can also decrease calcium absorption from the diet and increase the rate at which bone is lost. Therefore those taking this type of medication long-term will need to be mindful of its impact on bone health and take action to try and prevent osteoporosis.

Key dietary manipulation to help maintain bone health and prevent osteoporosis

The two nutrients that play a key role in bone health are calcium and vitamin D. Calcium is a major part of the structure of bones and vitamin D helps the body absorb calcium for the diet. Other vitamins and minerals play an important role too, so having a well-balanced, healthy diet is important for optimum bone health. Visit the National Osteoporosis Society website for more in-depth guidance on bone health at www.nos.org.uk or call their helpline on 0845 450 0230.

Taking nutritional supplements of calcium and vitamin D have been shown to improve bone density in RA sufferers taking corticosteroids. However, all those suffering joint and arthritic conditions, taking corticosteroids or not, should aim to consume sufficient calcium and vitamin D and try to promote and protect their bone health.

Try to:

- Stop smoking
- Get active-regular weight bearing activity like walking or dancing helps to promote bone strength
- Drink alcohol within the healthy recommendation of no more than 2–3 units a day for a woman and 3–4 for a man
- Avoid excessive intakes of caffeine
- Avoid eating too much salt. Current recommendations are 6g per day
- Avoid drinking a lot of fizzy drinks
- Have at least 700mg of calcium every day.

Many food manufacturers now put the calcium content on their products, making it easier to work out how much calcium will be in the portion.

Examples of calcium (mg) per portion:

> 1 pint of skimmed milk = 700mg
> 100ml low fat fruit yoghurt = 150mg
> 100g boiled spinach = 160mg
> 100g watercress = 170mg
> 2 dried figs = 200mg
> 3 dried apricots = 60mg
> 30g serving of fortified cereal (may vary) = 150mg. Served with skimmed milk (200ml) = a total of 400mg.

- Have sufficient vitamin D. The main source of vitamin D for the body is gathered from the action of sunlight on the skin-so get out and about in the sun, but be careful not to burn. 15–20 minutes in the sunlight, exposing the face and arms 3–4 times a week in the summer is thought to provide sufficient vitamin D for a healthy body. For those who are unable to get out and about in the sunlight, supplementation is recommended. Although dietary sources alone could not provide enough vitamin D the body needs, good sources include: fortified breakfast cereals, margarine, oily fish and egg yolk.

Methotrexate (MTX)

MTX is a powerful anti-inflammatory medication. MTX is also known to be a 'folate antagonist'. This means that it blocks the natural activity of folate. And, some research has found that people with RA tend to consume low levels of folate in their diets, further compounding this situation. Research into people who are on MTX, show that folate stores are lower than the general population too.

Folate, a naturally occurring vitamin (also called folic acid), is needed for the growth and repair of body cells. A folate deficiency can lead to a certain type of anaemia called 'megaloblastic anaemia' and has been shown to increase the risk of cardiovascular disease.

Megaloblastic anaemia

Red blood cells that carry oxygen around the bloodstream are produced in bone marrow. If red blood cells are not healthy, it reduces their capacity to carry oxygen around the body and this can have wide spread negative effects.

Megaloblastic anaemia is a condition that affects the healthy development of red blood cells within the bone marrow, leaving them enlarged and unable to perform their function effectively. This type of anaemia is caused by a deficiency in folate or vitamin B12. It is important to test for vitamin B12 deficiency before starting folate supplementation to make sure the right deficiency is identified and treated. Consult a qualified health professional for guidance.

Supplementing the diet with a modest dose of folate has been shown to reduce some side effects of MTX treatment. Supplementation at high levels has no shown any benefits. Ensuring a regular intake of folate rich foods is advisable for all those suffering joint and arthritic conditions, but in particular those on MTX. Folate rich foods include: yeast extract, liver, green leafy vegetables, oranges, pulses and fortified breakfast cereals.

Caffeine and MXT

It may be advisable to avoid caffeine when taking this medication. This is because caffeine belongs to a family of chemicals that can interfere with the effects of MTX, potentially reducing its effectiveness. There can be a wide variation in caffeine content of foods and drinks, so check the label of specific brands. Brewing time, water temperature and water content can affect caffeine levels too. Average caffeine contents per 200ml serving:

- Tea from a bag: 65mg
- Instant coffee: 60mg
- Filter coffee: 105mg

- Cola Dink: 50mg
- Energy drinks: 60mg
- 50g chocolate bar: 20mg

Avoiding: tea, coffee, cola, coca products and any other caffeine containing foods and drinks may help to maximise the medication's impact. If total avoidance is unrealistic, limiting intakes to less than 120mg a day could also help.

Dietary techniques to manage some common side effects of medications

Techniques to help with loss of taste or changes in taste:

- Foods that are strong in flavour may be preferred– choose stronger flavours of enjoyed foods like a stronger cheese.
- Sauces, seasoning, gravy, herbs, marinades, pickles and spices can all help to add extra taste to food.
- Experiment with different foods and tastes.
- Avoid very cold or hot foods.
- If meat tastes bitter, try soaking in wine, soya sauce or fruit juices to help minimise this taste.
- If meat tastes bitter, try avoiding foods sweetened with saccharine, as this may exacerbate this taste.
- Clearing the palate with a glass of water with lemon juice in it before eating can help to enhance taste.
- Drink refreshing drinks such as herbal teas, orange juice or lemonade.
- Keep the mouth and teeth clean.
- Rinse or brush teeth before eating.
- Use toothpaste that is non-mint flavour – this may help to reduce aberrant taste in the mouth.

- Try using a spray mister before and during meals.
- If a metallic taste is present; try using plastic or glass utensils.
- If a metallic or bitter taste is present; try sucking on sugar free mints, lemon drops or chewing gum.

1. Make a list of all the foods that have been affected by changes in taste.
2. For each food, try to think of the following;
   a. Are there any suitable alternatives that are of similar nutritional content. For example if the taste of red meat is affected, try replacing with poultry, fish, eggs, lentils, pulses or chesses.
   b. Can the taste be improved by marinating, adding sauces, spices or seasoning.
3. Make a list of anything that is needed to help with changes in taste, for example; non-mint toothpaste, spray mister, glass cutlery.

Techniques to help with nausea

- Try to eat 'little and often' having small meals and snacks – Instead of 3 meals a day, try to eat every 2–3 hours or have 6 small meals a day.
- Try to eat sitting down and sit in an upright position. Try not to lie down shortly after eating.
- Try to eat slowly.
- Try to avoid foods that have a strong smell.
- Cold foods may be better tolerated than hot foods.
- Plain, dry foods may be tolerated well.
- Try to avoid drinking half an hour before and during a meal.

- Try to avoid foods that are spicy.
- Try to avoid foods that are fatty.
- Try foods that are salty as they may help ease nausea.
- Try foods that contain ginger as they may help ease nausea, for example ginger biscuits, ginger beer, ginger ale and ginger tea.
- Getting some fresh air before eating may help.
- Eating food in a well-aired room can help to ease nausea.
- Anti-sickness medications can help – make sure they are taken as directed, as taking a regular dose if directed, even when not feeling nauseous, may help to improve effectiveness.
- Try to sips fluids throughout the day, as large volumes of fluid may increase nausea.

Sample menu using techniques to help with nausea:

Breakfast	A small cup of ginger tea
	2 small plain biscuits
Mid morning	A small glass of fruit juice
	A small pot of plain fat free yoghurt
Lunch	A bowl of soup and a slice of soft bread dipped in.
Mid afternoon	A small glass of a fizzy pop
	2 breadsticks dipped low fat soft cheese

Dinner	A gentle walk or spend some time in the garden
	Chilled pasta with tomatoes and olives
Evening snack	A small glass of sugar free squash
	2 ginger biscuits

Techniques to help with indigestion and heartburn

- Try to maintain a healthy weight: being overweight can make heartburn and indigestion symptoms worse.
- Have smaller, more frequent meals rather than 3 larger meals over the day. Eating little and often may help ease symptoms.
- Eat sitting up and eat slowly.
- Chew food well.
- Sip fluids during meals and snacks.
- Try to avoid eating or drinking 3–4 hours before going to bed.
- Try to avoid caffeine and alcohol.
- Try to avoid rich fatty foods.
- Try to avoid spicy foods.

Useful Charities

National Rheumatoid Arthritis Society
www.rheumatoid.org.uk
Call – 0800 298 7650

Arthritis Care
www.arthritiscare.org.uk
Call – 0808 800 4050

Arthritis Research Campaign (ARC)
www.arc.org.uk
Call – 0870 850 5000

Disabled living foundation
www.dlf.org.uk
Call – 0845 130 9177

The National Osteoporosis Society
www.nos.org.uk
Call – 0845 450 0230

Index

About the Author

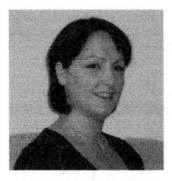

Zoe Hellman Bsc SRD is a State Registered Dietitian and has worked in the public and private sectors. She firmly believes in the importance of nutrition and the impact it can have on well-being and health. This is her second book and she brings her considerable experience to bear, in the hope that those affected by joint and arthritic conditions may benefit.

For more information on this book, and other books in the emerald series, go to: www.emeraldpublishing.co.uk